# BEAT PMT
# THROUGH DIET

*'No illness which can be treated by diet should be treated by any other means.'*

Maimonides      twelfth-century physician

# BEAT PMT
# THROUGH DIET

*The Women's Nutritional Advisory Service Programme based on medically proven treatment*

Maryon Stewart

*with contributions from* Dr Alan Stewart and Dr Guy Abraham

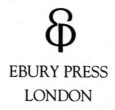

EBURY PRESS
LONDON

*To daughters everywhere*

## IMPORTANT NOTE FOR SUFFERERS

There are many fairly technical terms used to describe the Pre-Menstrual Syndrome and the normal menstrual cycle. You may already be familiar with some of the more technical terms, whilst others will be new to you. I have prepared a brief Dictionary of Terms to refer to which begins on page 221. Please don't be afraid to use it as often as necessary. The better you understand the information, the more you will be able to apply it to your own life and symptoms.

If your symptoms occur at other times of the month, apart from during your pre-menstrual time, you should have a medical check-up with your own doctor. If your symptoms are very severe it would be advisable to have your nutritional programme supervised by your own doctor or a trained counsellor. If you get confused or need extra advice, the Women's Nutritional Advisory Service is there to help you. All letters receive a personal reply: their address is on page 228.

Published by Ebury Press
Random Century House
20 Vauxhall Bridge Road
London SW1V 2SA

First Impression 1987
Reprinted 1988
Reprinted 1989 (twice)
Revised edition 1990
Reprinted 1991

Text copyright © 1987 and 1990 by Maryon Stewart, Dr Alan Stewart, Dr Guy Abraham

Foreword copyright © 1987 by Leslie Kenton

Illustrations copyright © 1987 by Mike Gordon

ISBN 0 85223 862 2

Designed by Gwyn Lewis
Edited by Suzanne Webber and Sarah Thomson
Illustrations by Mike Gordon

Computerset by MFK Typesetting Ltd, Hitchin, Herts.
Printed and bound in Great Britain by Mackays of Chatham PLC, Chatham, Kent.

# CONTENTS

Foreword by Leslie Kenton     7

Introduction     9

PART ONE     THE REALITIES OF PMT
Chapter 1     A problem as old as the hills     11
Chapter 2     Functioning normally     14
Chapter 3     PMT defined     21
Chapter 4     The making of PMT     24
Chapter 5     Anxious, irritable and uptight     28
Chapter 6     Bloating, weight gain and breast tenderness     49
Chapter 7     Sugar cravings, headaches and fatigue     56
Chapter 8     Depression, crying and thoughts of suicide     64
Chapter 9     Other symptoms – clumsiness, loss of sex drive and
                   agoraphobia     79
Chapter 10     The social implications of PMT     91

PART TWO     NUTRITION AND OUR BODIES
Chapter 11     Why is PMT more common today?     96
Chapter 12     A review of nutritional, drug and hormonal treatments     112
Chapter 13     Nutrition and the body: vitamins and minerals, what
                    they do     120

PART THREE     THE NUTRITIONAL APPROACH – A SELF-HELP MANUAL
Chapter 14     Choosing a nutritional plan     137
Chapter 15     Option 3 – A tailor-made nutritional programme     149
Chapter 16     Nutritious recipes     179
Chapter 17     Stress or distress?     195
Chapter 18     The value of exercise and relaxation     198
Chapter 19     Other valuable therapies     208
Chapter 20     Other nutritionally related problems     212
Chapter 21     Men who no longer suffer     217

PART FOUR     APPENDICES
1 Dictionary of terms 221     2 List of food additives 224     3 Organic and
specialized food suppliers 224     4 List of supplement stockists 225
5 Recommended reading list 226     6 Useful addresses 227     7 Substitutes for
excluded foods 230     8 Charts and diaries 231     9 References 234     Index 237

## ACKNOWLEDGEMENTS

I would like to acknowledge all the researchers that have gone before us who collectively have completed the groundwork that allowed us to begin our work from an advanced point. In particular I refer to the work of Dr Katharina Dalton, Dr Michael Brush, Dr David Horrobin and Dr Shaughn O'Brien. I would like to acknowledge the work of Dr Guy Abraham and Dr Alan Stewart. Without their technical support we would not have been able to provide such valuable help to so many women, and education on the nutritional approach to the Pre-Menstrual Syndrome to so many doctors and medical organizations.

My heartfelt thanks also go to all the patients who have volunteered to share their case histories with us in this book. Their willingness to divulge intimate details so frankly in an effort to help others is highly appreciated.

Special mentions are due to three valued helpers. Dr Alan Stewart and Dr Guy Abraham have been a constant technical support since the Advisory Service began. Sarah Tooley, our Senior Nurse, has been my right arm for the last six years and has given me much support with this book.

My thanks must also go to the caring and efficient team at the Women's Nutritional Advisory Service. Without them this book would never have been possible.

I would also like to thank Julia Swift for her advice on exercise, Deryn Bell for her advice on osteopathy and Paul Lundberg for his advice on acupuncture and acupressure.

Finally, I would like to thank my wonderful little children, Phoebe, Chesney and Hester, who kept me going with their cuddles when I most needed them.

*Maryon Stewart*

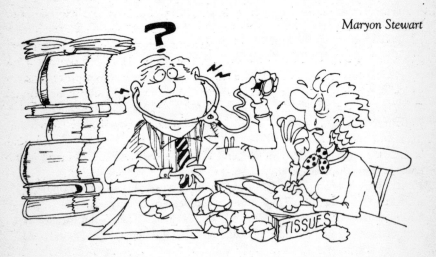

# FOREWORD
# BY
# LESLIE KENTON

This is an extraordinary book. Not only does it tackle the very complex subject of Pre-Menstrual Syndrome (PMT) in a simple and straightforward way so that it becomes understandable to the average woman suffering from it, but it is also eminently practical. It tells you exactly how to go about finding the answer to your own difficulties.

PMT, with its symptoms of bloating, depression, irritability, fatigue and all the rest is not something 'normal' which you have to suffer from, month in month out. I have seen even the most resistant cases turn around through changes of diet, alterations in living habits and the judicious use of certain nutritional supplements. What Maryon Stewart has done so cleverly is to explain how to help yourself: first by making you aware of what your specific problems are, and then by helping you outline a self-directed lifestyle programme for solving them.

And Maryon Stewart can substantiate her claims too. Having already put into practice the natural approach to PMT set out in this book for six years, and having monitored its results on a thousand women through the Women's Nutritional Advisory Service, she knows what she is talking about. The methods work. And her advice about eating natural organically-grown foods, using simple techniques which can help you better manage stress, calling on well-planned nutritional supplements when necessary and even making use of natural treatments which you can carry out yourself to cope with acute problems is not only sound in relation to eliminating PMT. It can also be taken far beyond to form the basis of a total lifestyle for optimum health for women and men alike. *Beat PMT Through Diet* is a book to be read, used and then loaned to friends when they need it.

**Maryon Stewart** studied preventive dentistry and nutrition at the Royal Dental Hospital in London and worked as a counsellor with nutritional doctors in England for four years. She set up the Women's Nutritional Advisory Service (formerly the PMT Advisory Service) at the beginning of 1984 to bring nutritional help to all women sufferers of this under-acknowledged condition. Under her direction, the Women's Nutritional Advisory Service has provided help to women all over the world, a medical information service for doctors and other health workers, and a clinical trials unit. In February 1987 she launched the Women's Nutritional Advisory Service which now provides broader help to women. Maryon is married to Dr Alan Stewart. They have three children.

**Dr Alan Stewart** qualified from Guy's Hospital, London, in 1976 and spent five years specializing in hospital medicine. He became a member of the Royal College of Physicians (MRCP UK). For the last ten years he has had a major interest in nutrition, and is a founding member of, and Information Officer of the British Society for Nutritional Medicine. He is also Medical Advisor to the Women's Nutritional Advisory Service.

**Guy E. Abraham, MD,** is a former Professor of Obstetrics and Gynaecological Endocrinology at UCLA School of Medicine. Because of his research over the past 18 years on the development of sophisticated techniques to measure minute quantities of hormones in blood, he has received worldwide recognition: the General Diagnostic Award of the Canadian Association of Clinical Chemists in 1974; the Medaille d'Honneur of the University of Liège, Belgium, 1976; the Senior Investigator Award of the Clinical Radiossay Society in 1980. The applications of these techniques to various female disorders have improved markedly the understanding of these disorders and their management. He is the Patron of the Women's Nutritional Advisory Service.

# INTRODUCTION

The Pre-Menstrual Syndrome, or PMT, does not have the physical characteristics of an abscess or an ingrown toenail. Neither does it show up under a microscope like a diseased cell. The agony and the anguish suffered, not to mention the misery and the mental torture, cannot easily be measured.

Perhaps because PMT is relatively difficult to detect or quantify by an outsider the condition has taken far longer than it should have done to become recognized, and still longer to be treated effectively without the use of drugs. As a result, women have had to go on suffering unnecessarily.

> 'My doctor told me it was all in my mind. But I gain five inches (12 cm) pre-menstrually around the middle. I told him indignantly that if it was anywhere it was all in the waist!'

> 'My monthly symptoms were diagnosed as "problems with my nerves". I was prescribed tranquillizers which I became too dependent upon.'

> 'I was told by my doctor that the solution to my symptoms is to have a baby. I'm single, I don't have a regular boyfriend, and I don't want a baby!'

> 'All part of being a woman' is a hot favourite, followed by 'PMT symptoms are a sign of a woman rejecting her femininity'.

The most inventive advice for overcoming PMT symptoms was the treatment prescribed by a doctor who advised his patient to join the Conservative Party and become a magistrate, as his wife had done previously!

To a non-sufferer this may sound amusing. However, to a woman with PMT who is feeling wretched, in some cases suicidal, and certainly bitter that her life is being disrupted by this condition, it is really no laughing matter.

There exists now a wealth of evidence to show that PMT not only exists, but that it can be treated, to a large degree, quite naturally. The reason why this approach is not widely recognized is that the medical research on PMT has hitherto been scattered far and wide in medical journals around the world. By gathering this information together we were able to formulate a very simple, effective programme to help overcome Pre-Menstrual Syndrome.

In order to make this often life-saving information available to anyone and everyone in need, the Women's Nutritional Advisory Service was set up as an interim measure. For six years we have been helping thousands of women, not only in Britain, but indeed all over the world.

The Women's Nutritional Advisory Service has carried out a scientific survey of the symptoms, progress and treatment of 1000 women who have consulted them. Throughout the book you will find figures and charts which refer to this survey, unless stated otherwise, as for example, when particular studies were made of individual cases and groups.

We have also been able to provide a Medical Information Service which regularly supplies doctors and other health care professionals with information about the nutritional approach to PMT. The ideal situation is that the nutritional approach to PMT becomes recognized as a valid part of orthodox medicine and is practised widely.

In the meantime, this book has been put together based on a very successful programme which the Women's Nutritional Advisory Service has been using for the last six years. I have hard facts to substantiate our claims, as you will see as you read on. The good news is that overcoming PMT consists mainly of SELF-HELP with a little education along the way.

The book will explain to you how you can solve the problem for yourself, according to your own individual symptoms. It is written in four parts. Part One deals with the realities of Pre-Menstrual Tension and the effect it has on individual and family life. Part Two covers nutrition in relation to our body. Part Three is devoted to diet and other means of self-help, and finally, in Part Four, you will find lists of useful information and addresses.

Consider your voyage through this book an adventure, and as we often say to the sufferers beginning our programme – 'May you never be the same again!'

Good Luck!

# 1

# A PROBLEM
# AS OLD AS
# THE HILLS

Despite the fact that for the last few years we have been talking and writing about the Pre-Menstrual Syndrome (PMT) as if it has just been discovered, in reality it has been affecting women all over the world for many years.

I am often asked the question 'How come PMT is more common now than it was years ago?' My answer is that we talk about the condition far more now than we used to, and that our twentieth-century diet may well be making matters worse.

The whole event has become affectionately nicknamed 'The Curse'. It seems that this term derives from ancient times when a menstruating woman was considered by society to be unclean, and in some cases dangerous. In some primitive tribes menstrual blood was considered to be evil, and a menstruating woman had to remain shut away for fear that she would cast a spell on the menfolk or kill off whole herds of animals using her temporary 'witch's' powers. If a menstruating woman disobeyed this or similar rules and mixed with the menfolk, some tribes would even condemn her to death.

Certain religions still regard a menstruating woman as undesirable. In the Moslem religion a menstruating woman is not allowed to enter the mosque. As recently as the beginning of this century a Greek Orthodox woman was not permitted Communion during her period, and to this day in the Orthodox Jewish religion, menstruating women are not permitted to sleep with their husbands during their period.

Is it any wonder that complexes about the whole subject developed and that the subject became taboo? Who, with any degree of sanity, would have wanted to admit the fact that their period was due? It makes the mind boggle!

Despite the fact that women's often frenzied accounts of their unbearable pre-menstrual symptoms have been labelled as being 'all in the mind', i.e. a mental condition, past treatments included hysterectomies, electric shock treatment, and even, in tragic cases, lobotomies (an operation where part of the brain is removed).

It seems there have been several dilemmas. Firstly whether PMT actually exists or not, and secondly, assuming it does exist, is it a physical condition or a mental condition? Traditionally, Western medicine tends to regard a physical condition as one that we have no control over, and a mental condition as one that is self-perpetuated.

The first recorded cases of PMT were in 1931, when Dr Robert T. Frank, an American physician working in New York reported 15 cases of Pre-Menstrual Tension. These women had symptoms of nervous tension, water retention and weight gain. Dr Frank found a high level of the hormone oestrogen present in these patients and felt that they were unable to excrete the oestrogen from their bodies pre-menstrually. The excess oestrogen, he felt, then irritated the nervous system, and thus symptoms developed.

Further work was done by other American doctors in this field. In 1938 Dr Israel, another American doctor, presented his theory that not all women had high levels of oestrogen, but they did have low levels of the hormone progesterone.

In 1943 Dr Biskind published a study which supported the theory that many pre-menstrual symptoms reported were similar to vitamin B deficiency symptoms. He found that treatment with vitamin B greatly improved symptoms, especially uncomfortable breast symptoms and heavy bleeding during menstruation, which are also symptoms of vitamin B deficiency. The cause was an overload of oestrogen pre-menstrually.

As early as 1944 Dr Harris observed women with pre-menstrual fatigue, nervousness and cravings for sweet foods. Further research along these lines continued in the 1950s.

In 1953 Dr Katharina Dalton, a British doctor, began publishing her work. She and Dr Raymond Greene renamed the condition 'Pre-Menstrual Syndrome', as they identified so many symptoms as being pre-menstrual. Dr Dalton is considered a pioneer in this field. She spent many years identifying the magnitude of the problem in prisons, hospitals, factories, offices and schools. She also studied the relationship between pre-menstrual symptoms and crime, alcoholism and drug abuse. Quite a few of her studies are mentioned later on in the text, as they served as a starting point for our own research. Dr Dalton supports the theory that pre-menstrually low levels of the hormone progesterone are present. Her treatment consists largely of progesterone supplementation.

Since 1972 Dr Guy Abraham has researched the subject of PMT in depth. He has published many medical papers on the nutritional approach to PMT. During the course of his research he classified four different sub-groups of PMT. He worked out a treatment plan for each different sub-group, thus helping other doctors to recognise and treat the condition. We have used Dr Abraham's classifications throughout the book.

The nutritional approach to treatment is favoured as it is natural, and does not involve taking drugs or hormones. Many experts now agree that it is the best first-line treatment for PMT.

As you have probably gathered, despite the fact that the Pre-Menstrual Syndrome has been approached from many angles, confusion still exists on the subject. There are those schools who believe the condition should be treated with hormones, whilst others believe it is a psychological condition which should be treated with tranquillizers and anti-depressants.

As a group we haven't set out to prove whether it is in fact a physical or mental condition. *We know it is a real condition.* Instead, we approach it from the viewpoint that certain symptoms exist which may be overcome by making dietary changes and adjustments in lifestyles where necessary. Between us we have many years of experience and have been able to help tens of thousands of women around the world to overcome their pre-menstrual problems.

I aim to give you a good understanding of what happens to your body during your monthly cycle. I will then help you to identify what the symptoms may be due to and then, of course, how you can go about getting them sorted out.

# 2

# FUNCTIONING NORMALLY

## THE NORMAL MENSTRUAL CYCLE

In order to understand what is going wrong with your menstrual cycle, it is important to have a fairly good understanding of what the normal menstrual cycle is.

The age at the onset of periods has been decreasing at a rate of three years per century. Periods begin between the tenth and sixteenth year in 95 per cent of European girls, and between the tenth and fifteenth year in American girls. The age at the onset of the menopause, when periods cease, has been increasing at a rate of three years per century as well. Menopause occurs between the ages of 40 and 55.

The menstrual cycle is a fertility cycle, a fascinating process that enables a woman to conceive a child. This cycle is repeated each month, and if fertilization does not occur the cycle ends with a menstrual period – the shedding of the lining of the womb in preparation for the next cycle. The cycle can vary in length from approximately 22 days up to 34 days. Anything between these numbers would be considered normal. The first day of bleeding, the day the period arrives, is referred to as the first day of the cycle.

## THE ORGANS INVOLVED

There are specific organs which each play an important role in the menstrual cycle. They are designed to work together so that a woman can become pregnant and nourish the growing child throughout the nine months of pregnancy.

14

The uterus or womb, as it is more commonly known, is a hollow, pear-shaped, muscular organ which is about three inches (7.5 cm) long in a non-pregnant woman. There are many layers of specialized muscle here which, as if by magic, can expand so that the uterus becomes many times its usual size during pregnancy. The growing child lives in the uterus until it is ready to be born.

The innermost layer of the uterus is a membrane called the endometrium. During the cycle it becomes filled with the blood supply which would be needed to nourish a pregnancy. If conception has not occurred the endometrium breaks down, and together with the blood leaves the uterus through the neck of the uterus, which is known as the cervix.

The cervix or neck of the womb is like a little ball towards the back of the vagina. It has a small opening which remains closed for most of the time. A few days before the egg is released by the ovary, the cervix begins to open. By the time the egg has left the ovary, the opening would have become wide enough to let the sperm swim up through it, in order to gain access to the egg.

For a few days each cycle, at the time of ovulation, the specialized cells in the cervix produce fertile cervical mucus, which allows the sperm to live during their journey to the uterus. At other times during the menstrual cycle the cervix produces infertile cervical mucus which prevents the sperm from surviving.

Once the menstrual blood passes through the cervix it flows into the vaginal canal, a four- to six-inch (10–15 cm) muscular tube which has the ability to widen during sexual intercourse and during labour. During intercourse the lining of the vaginal canal becomes engorged with blood. A slippery liquid is produced which is designed to make the experience of sexual intercourse more comfortable.

The two almond-shaped organs on either side of the uterus are called the ovaries. They contain thousands of immature eggs which are present in a baby girl even before birth! From puberty, usually, one egg will leave one ovary during each menstrual cycle. I say usually, as there are occasions when more than one egg becomes fertilized simultaneously, and multiple births result.

## OVULATION

The process of the egg leaving the ovary is called ovulation. At about 12 to 16 days before menstruation, the ovary will release an egg. The egg is then usually picked up by one of the Fallopian tubes, which is where the egg and the sperm would meet if conception were to take place. The Fallopian tubes are a pair of very thin tubes, about four inches (10 cm) long, which are connected to each side to the uterus. The egg waits for the sperm in the Fallopian tube for between 12 and 24 hours. If no sperm arrive, the egg is then absorbed by the body. If the egg and the sperm do meet and join up, fertilization takes place, and the fertilized egg will then move down, over the next few days, into the uterus, where it becomes embedded in the lining. This fertilized egg then grows into a baby.

## WHAT CONTROLS THE CYCLE?

It is important to understand that although we have looked at the various organs at work for us during the menstrual cycle, it is actually the brain that controls the ovaries. In fact, a particular part of the brain called the pituitary gland sends instructions to the ovaries to make them function. The pituitary gland will tell the ovaries when to produce eggs and release them. It also stimulates production by the ovaries of oestrogen and progesterone, two very special sex hormones. If no fertilization occurs, the pituitary gland will send a new signal for the ovaries to begin producing eggs again.

## WHAT ACTUALLY HAPPENS DURING THE CYCLE?

Either just prior to your period arriving, or during your period, several eggs will begin to grow in the ovary. Each egg is surrounded by a sac which is called a follicle. The egg and the follicle grow together. The follicle produces oestrogen which, as you can see from the chart below, is at its highest during the latter part of the first half of the cycle. Oestrogen is responsible for the production of fertile cervical mucus, the opening of the cervix to allow the sperm in to meet the eggs, and the building up of blood in the lining of the uterus, preparing for a fertilized egg.

The cervical mucus is usually very fertile indeed: it is reckoned that sperm can survive for as long as five days in the fertile cervical mucus, waiting for an egg to fertilize. The egg is released from the ovary anything from eight to 14 days from the first day of your cycle – the day your period begins. Ovulation tends to vary from person to person. Some women are aware that they are ovulating as they experience some short-lived pain or stinging sensations in the area of the right or left ovary.

The cells or follicle that protected the egg before it was released remain in the ovary after the egg has left. The follicle develops into a special gland known as the corpus luteum. Whereas the cells of the follicle were producing large amounts of oestrogen during the first half of the cycle, after ovulation they begin to produce the other important sex hormone, progesterone.

Progesterone is an important hormone at the beginning of pregnancy as it is responsible for producing infertile mucus, preventing sperm and other substances from harming a pregnancy. It is sometimes known as the pregnancy protecting

16

## THE NORMAL MENSTRUAL CYCLE

1
2
   *Period begins – lining of uterus comes away. Very little progesterone. Very little oestrogen.*

3
4
5
6
7
   *Eggs growing and follicles beginning to produce oestrogen.*

   *Oestrogen levels rising.*

8
9
10
11
12
13
   *Oestrogen levels high, stimulating the lining of the uterus to thicken.*

14
15
   *Ovulation occurs approximately at this time. Oestrogen levels are high. Once the egg has left, the follicle begins producing progesterone.*

16
17
18
19
20
21
22
23
24
25
   *Oestrogen and progesterone levels high.*

26
27
28
   *Both progesterone and oestrogen levels falling now that conception has not occurred.*

hormone. It also closes the cervix and holds the lining of the uterus in place from ovulation until the next period begins, if fertilization has not taken place. Progesterone levels are sometimes low in women who suffer with PMT, and it has been demonstrated that balancing a woman's nutritional condition can raise the levels of progesterone again. This will be discussed later in the section on nutritional supplements on page 174.

After ovulation the body waits to see whether a pregnancy has occurred. Once it realizes that pregnancy has not occurred, the corpus luteum of the ovary stops working, and the levels of both oestrogen and progesterone fall. As progesterone has been holding the lining of the uterus in place, when this hormone level drops the lining of the uterus is then shed and a menstrual period occurs.

## THE MAIN FACTS

Oestrogen controls the first half of the cycle until the egg leaves the ovary, and progesterone is in control of the cycle from the day the egg is released until the menstrual period begins.

The hormones produced by the ovaries have a profound effect on moods and behaviour – not surprising, since oestrogen is a stimulant of the nervous system. Low oestrogen levels cause depression, whereas high oestrogen levels can result in symptoms such as anxiety, irritability and nervous tension. The correct amount of oestrogen produces assertiveness, motivation and emotional stability. Progesterone, on the other hand, is a depressant, and has a calming effect. It is therefore obvious that for a woman to function normally throughout the menstrual cycle a proper balance of these hormones must be maintained.

I will be talking more about how the levels of oestrogen and progesterone are affected by a deficient nutritional state in Chapter 13 on vitamins and minerals, and our laboratory findings. Although it was previously thought that a woman had to take supplements of hormones in order to maintain her levels if she was deficient, it appears that this is not always so, as you will see.

## EFFECTS OF NUTRITION
## ON THE MENSTRUAL CYCLE

Nutrition affects the menstrual cycle in many ways. First, there are certain nutrients such as amino acids and vitamins that are necessary for the manufacture of brain hormones and the normal function of the pituitary gland, and which are also capable of influencing moods and behaviour.

Hormones are produced by the ovaries, adrenal glands and the thyroid gland.

18

As already noted, the ovaries produce the sex hormones, oestrogen and progesterone. The adrenal glands produce both sex hormones and hormones related to stress. The thyroid gland produces its own hormones that control the body's rate of metabolism. These three glands – the ovaries, adrenals and thyroid – are all in turn controlled by a part of the brain, the pituitary which, if you like, is the conductor of the hormonal orchestra. It in turn is sensitive to a part of the brain called the hypothalamus which also influences appetite, temperature control and the 24-hour 'biological clock' that controls our eating and sleeping rhythms. It also contains another 'clock' that controls the 28-day menstrual cycle. Finally, it in turn is influenced by levels of stress and emotion. Thus it is that external stress and emotional factors can influence hormonal factors, and ultimately, one's physical sense of well-being and mood.

When an imbalanced diet exists or there are nutritional deficiencies the whole system may become disturbed or more sensitive. If there is a severe reduction in calorie (kj) intake and the body weight falls to an unhealthy level, the function of

## HOW YOUR HORMONAL SYSTEM WORKS

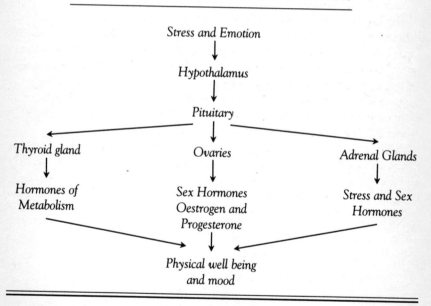

Stress and Emotion

Hypothalamus

Pituitary

Thyroid gland

Hormones of
Metabolism

Ovaries

Sex Hormones
Oestrogen and
Progesterone

Adrenal Glands

Stress and Sex
Hormones

Physical well being
and mood

the pituitary gland will decrease and periods may cease altogether, or may continue but without ovulation. This is nature's way of protecting a woman from becoming pregnant when in an unhealthy state – a rather drastic form of contraception!

A balance of vitamin B6 and zinc may be of great importance to some of the biochemical reactions that occur in the region of the hypothalamus and pituitary. Zinc may also influence the metabolism of thyroid hormones. The adrenal glands characteristically contain the highest concentration of vitamin C of any part of the body. So ensuring an adequate supply of these vitamins and minerals is probably crucial in maintaining a healthy hormonal balance.

Finally, physical and emotional stress can have a powerful effect upon the menstrual cycle. For example, excessive or severe physical exercise, if continued on a regular basis, may cause the pituitary to 'switch off' the ovaries. Thus periods cease and the level of the sex hormone oestrogen may fall. Such women put themselves at risk of fractures and thinning of the bones – osteoporosis. Emotional stress, such as the worry of becoming pregnant from having unprotected sexual intercourse, can itself lead to the delay or the missing of a period, which in turn causes increased worry and stress – not an uncommon experience at some time in one's life.

So a healthy diet and the avoidance of physical and mental stresses play an important part in health, and especially in the control of Pre-Menstrual Tension.

# 3

# PMT DEFINED

PMT, or Pre-Menstrual Syndrome, as it is more correctly known, is the term used to describe a collection of physical and mental symptoms that occur before a period starts and cease with or shortly after the arrival of a period.

## WHEN DO SYMPTOMS BEGIN AND END?

- Most commonly symptoms begin from a week to a few days before menstruation begins, and then diminish as the period begins.

- Sometimes symptoms occur at the time of ovulation (mid cycle), then disappear until a few days pre-menstrually, when they recur until the onset of the period.

- Symptoms may begin at the time of ovulation, around the middle of the cycle, gradually increasing in severity until the period begins. It is not uncommon for symptoms to persist to the first day or two of the period.

## WHAT IS THE DIFFERENCE BETWEEN PRE-MENSTRUAL SYNDROME AND PRE-MENSTRUAL TENSION?

- Pre-Menstrual Tension was the original name given to the collection of symptoms relating to tension and anxiety first reported by Dr Frank in the 1930s. Thus the condition became known as 'PMT'.

- Further research was done, particularly by Dr Dalton, who went on to discover further types of symptoms. She renamed the condition Pre-Menstrual Syndrome (PMS).

- Although the condition this book is written about is technically Pre-Menstrual Syndrome, we came to realize some years ago that most women use its original name, PMT. For this reason alone we have chosen to use the term PMT.

- The term PMT in this book relates to all the symptoms described for the condition of Pre-Menstrual Syndrome.

## THE MOST COMMON PMT SYMPTOMS

Have a look at these symptoms. You might be surprised to realize that they are all associated with Pre-Menstrual Syndrome.

| | | | |
|---|---|---|---|
| Nervous tension | Agoraphobia | Hayfever | Thoughts of |
| Mood swings | Bad breath | Fatigue | suicide |
| Irritability | Sensitivity to | Confusion | Sensitivity to |
| Anxiety | light | Forgetfulness | noise |
| Depression | Disorientation | Crying | Excessive thirst |
| Headache | Restlessness | Dizziness | Hostility |
| Migraine | Mouth ulcers | Tremors and | Sugar cravings |
| Insomnia | Acne | shakes | |
| | | | |
| Swollen breasts | Backache | Fainting | Weight gain |
| Tender/sore breasts | Heart poundings | Asthma | |
| | | | |
| Swollen abdomen | Cramp pains | Loss of interest in | Diarrhoea |
| Bloated feelings | Wind | sex | Cystitis |
| Craving for food | Generalized aches | Constipation | |
| | | | |
| Swelling of | Increased physical | Clumsiness | Boils |
| extremities | activity | Eczema | Hives |
| | | | |
| Heavy aching legs | Restless legs | Painful joints | Swollen ankles |

## JUST KNOWING THAT IT IS PMT

We are often told by patients that just knowing they have an identifiable, not to mention treatable, condition brings much relief in itself. It was a real surprise to me initially to discover women in all walks of life, with varying educational backgrounds, who were under the impression that their symptoms were in one of the following categories:

- All part of being a woman.

- Part of the ageing process.

- Early senile dementia.

- A psychological problem.

- A character fault.

- Schizophrenia.

The chances are that you may have been under an illusion that you fit in to one of these categories. I have lost count of the numbers of women who describe themselves as 'Jekyll and Hyde', i.e. two quite separate people during their menstrual cycle. They all seem to be acutely aware of the change as it occurs some time after ovulation. To a woman, they feel quite powerless to overcome the symptoms.

## THE DIFFERENCE BETWEEN PMT AND PERIOD PAINS

| Characteristic | PMT | Period pains |
|---|---|---|
| 1. Time of onset | 3–14 days before period | One day before and/or on first day or two of period |
| 2. Improvement | Approximately the onset of the period | Some time during or at the end of the period |
| 3. After childbirth | Symptoms worsen | Symptoms improve |

# 4

# THE MAKING
# OF PMT

There are a number of factors that may cause or contribute to PMT symptoms. It is very important to examine these thoroughly in order to get the situation into perspective.

## GYNAECOLOGICAL OR HORMONAL PROBLEMS

If you have been experiencing problems for some time it is important to consult your doctor for a full check-up. Certainly if you have symptoms that are persistent all month through, there may be other complications present. Here is a small checklist for you to look at to see whether there need be cause for any concern:

- Heavy or irregular periods.

- Abdominal pain.

- Excessive weight gain or weight loss.

- Facial hair growth.

- Persistent severe headaches.

- Current vaginal discharge, soreness or irritation.

- Breast lumps or tenderness throughout the menstrual cycle.

- Milky discharge from the nipples.

If any of these are a current problem it would be advisable to get them checked out, for peace of mind if nothing else. You will then establish whether you have other medical problems as well as PMT, or pure PMT.

## FACTORS IN THE CAUSATION OF PMT

1. Difficulty with relationships.

2. Problems with work.

3. Problem children to cope with.

4. Disturbed night's sleep.

5. Financial difficulties causing friction and worries.

6. Strained relations with husband or partner.

7. Inadequate or incorrect diet.

8. Environmental pollutants.

9. Social poisons.

10. Oral contraceptive pill.

11. Increasing age, especially age 30–40.

12. After childbirth.

13. Lack of exercise.

14. Operations and physical illnesses.

## EXAMINING PMT SYMPTOMS

## WHAT ACTUALLY CAUSES PMT

In Chapter 2, 'Functioning Normally', hormonal changes throughout the menstrual cycle were described. Whilst major disturbance of hormone levels is not the sole explanation for PMT, certain variations in hormone levels or sensitivity to hormones may well be part of the cause. This in turn can be influenced by stress, dietary factors and nutritional state.

If you are confused about the cause of PMT, don't worry, as most medical scientists and researchers are just as perplexed. Dr Guy Abraham, former Professor of Obstetrics and Gynaecology at the University of California in Los Angeles, has attempted to unravel the causation of PMT by dividing the symptoms into four groups, as detailed below. This somewhat artificial classification does help us to develop possible explanations as to the cause of different aspects of PMT symptoms. Disturbances in the levels of oestrogen and progesterone have been described in some sufferers with different types of PMT, but these are not universal changes. Furthermore, many women will experience symptoms from more than one sub-group.

### PMT A (anxiety)

This is the most common sub-group. Symptoms are recorded in about 80 per cent of sufferers. The symptoms in this group are:

Nervous tension.
Mood swings.
Irritability.
Anxiety.

### PMT H (hydration)

This is the second sub-group. It is estimated that symptoms occur in 60 per cent of sufferers. The symptoms in the sub-group are as follows:

Weight gain.
Swelling of extremities.
Breast tenderness.
Abdominal bloating.

### PMT C (craving)

This is the third sub-group. Symptoms probably occur in 40 per cent of sufferers. There are six symptoms in this sub-group:

Headache.
Craving for sweets.
Increased appetite.
Heart pounding.
Fatigue.
Dizziness or fainting.

## PMT D (depression)

Of all four sub-groups, this is the one least commonly found on its own. Perhaps 20 per cent of sufferers have PMT D. There are five symptoms in this category:

Depression.
Forgetfulness.
Crying.
Confusion.
Insomnia.

Each group seems to have different factors involved, except that inadequate diet and stress can be common to all of them. Although some women only suffer with one sub-group of symptoms, it is just as common to be suffering from any combination of sub-groups at the same time. Many severe sufferers seem to have symptoms in all four sub-groups initially.

In the next four chapters I will examine in greater detail each one of these sub-groups of symptoms and look at how the symptoms affected the lives of some of the women who contacted the Women's Nutritional Advisory Service. Rather than describing how PMT might affect various aspects of your life, I decided that the subject might become more alive if it was talked about by sufferers themselves. I have selected patients whose symptoms span a broad spectrum of the Pre-Menstrual Syndrome. By looking into their lives you may well recognize familiar situations.

# 5

# ANXIOUS, IRRITABLE AND UPTIGHT

## PMT A (ANXIETY)

The main symptoms of PMT A are nervous tension, anxiety, irritability and mood swings, beginning as early as two weeks before the period and becoming progressively worse as the period approaches.

It is thought that elevated levels of oestrogen, or increased sensitivity to oestrogen, are present in PMT A. As oestrogen builds up through the monthly cycle it passes to the liver where it is broken down and excreted by the liver into the bowel in an inactive form. In order to achieve this process, optimum levels of vitamin B must be present. If a vitamin B deficiency exists, the liver may not be able to break down the oestrogen for it to be excreted. Furthermore, on a low fibre and high animal fats diet, the inert oestrogen can be changed to an active form and reabsorbed, leading to higher levels of this hormone. Lack of adequate fibre and vitamin B may be important in PMT A.

The next question is: How can high levels of oestrogen cause symptoms? It is thought that excess oestrogen causes an imbalance in brain chemicals. Too much of some stimulating brain chemicals is made (serotonin, adrenaline and noradrenaline), and too little dopamine is produced. Dopamine normally has a calming, soothing effect on the body. With these chemicals out of balance, it is likely that the person will begin to feel uptight, irritable and nervous and have mood swings. Other effects of this particular imbalance may also be drowsiness, water retention and inability to concentrate and perform. Adequate levels of vitamin B, particularly B6, and the mineral magnesium, are necessary for normal dopamine production (see Chapter 13, p. 128) and a relative lack of them may well contribute to symptoms.

An additional factor in PMT A is caffeine. Caffeine is a mild stimulant and is found in tea, coffee, cola-based drinks, some pain killers and to a small degree in chocolate. In small doses, one or two cups of coffee, it can serve as a useful mental stimulant: in higher amounts anxiety, irritability, depression, nervousness, tremulousness, headache and increased passage of urine can all occur. Difficulty in getting off to sleep is another side effect, particularly if large amounts of tea or coffee are consumed in the evening. The average cup of tea contains 50 to 100 mg of caffeine and coffee anything from 75 to 200 mg. A total intake of more than 500 mg a day can produce symptoms. This effect is particularly likely to occur in women. Interestingly though, the hormone oestrogen reduces the rate of breakdown of caffeine in the body. An increase in sensitivity to caffeine can therefore occur during pregnancy. A combination of a high intake of caffeine and high circulating levels of oestrogen could well contribute to PMT A symptoms.

From a survey in *Fitness* magazine in 1987 the level of PMT symptoms in general seemed to relate to intake of tea and coffee. Similar findings have been observed in female workers in a Chinese tea processing plant.

A final and important factor is hyperventilation. This mouthful simply means over breathing. Often when one becomes anxious it is natural to increase the rate and depth of respiration. This provides more oxygen to the bloodstream but also removes more of the waste gas carbon dioxide. This lack of carbon dioxide causes a change in body chemistry which can actually aggravate or cause a variety of symptoms, including numbness and tingling of the fingers, hands and around the mouth, muscle cramps, headaches, light-headedness, increased anxiety, physical and mental fatigue and confusion. The solution is to relax, reduce the rate and depth of breathing and if symptoms are severe to breathe in and out of a paper bag for several minutes. Where these symptoms chronically occur, formal advice and breathing exercises may need to be given by a physiotherapist or psychologist.

## ABOUT THE SYMPTOMS

The symptoms in PMT A can at least be disturbing, and at worst feel like a tidal wave of personality change. They are amongst the most common symptoms in PMT.

A staggering 97 per cent of women in our scientific study complained that they suffered to some degree with irritability pre-menstrually, 73 per cent of them with severe irritability, 96 per cent reported mood swings, 62 per cent severe, while 95 per cent reported nervous tension, 60 per cent severe, and 91 per cent reported anxiety, 54 per cent severe.

| Degree of irritability suffered out of a sample of 1000 women | | | | |
|---|---|---|---|---|
| Not Affected | Mild | Moderate | Severe | Total Affected |
| 2.5% | 3.2% | 20.8% | 73.5% - | 97.5% |

As you can imagine, the implications of these figures are fairly devastating. No wonder so many women report Jekyll and Hyde syndrome! Let us look more closely at how PMT A affected the lives of some of our patients.

## PMT HITS HOME!

Many women were also reporting wild feelings of violence and aggression premenstrually. Their nervous tension seemed to reach uncontrollable peaks, at which time they would lash out at children and husbands or boyfriends. To a woman, they reported that this behaviour was uncharacteristic of them, and that it was having disastrous effects on their families.

The chart below shows to what degree violent and aggressive feelings were a problem. We were very concerned indeed by the result of our research.

Just under 80 per cent of the women studied felt violent or aggressive premenstrually. This obviously had serious repercussions on their partners, and on their children in particular.

| Sample of 1000 women who admitted being violent/aggressive whilst suffering from PMT | | | | |
|---|---|---|---|---|
| Not Affected | Once | More Than Once | More Than Six Times | Total Affected |
| 20.6% | 4.7% | 27.7% | 47.0% - | 79.4% |

## " Pauline's Story* "

Pauline experienced extreme violent and aggressive feelings pre-menstrually. She actually used to strike her husband and her daughter. She relates her experiences here very frankly.

Pauline is a 35-year-old mother and housewife who has had PMT since she was 13 years old.

*'I used to be able to cope when I was in my teens but as I became older, my symptoms became really dreadful. I used to feel groggy for the whole week before my period. I had terrible migraine headaches and my head felt like it was full of cotton wool. Towards the end I'd have to spend the last few days in bed as I had no energy. I also had severe insomnia, dizziness and forgetfulness.*

*Eventually I started hitting my one-year-old daughter. I knew it was wrong but I couldn't control myself. I even hit my husband. I tried to carry on with life pre-menstrually but the very thought of going out of the house sent me into fits of the shakes. I was very frightened of meeting people. In fact, I was terrified!*

*I was given so many treatments for PMT. First my doctor prescribed different types of pill. Then I had Valium and I wasn't sleeping. That's when the depression started. Then I had anti-depressants. I felt like a junkie with my "uppers and downers".*

*Hormone treatment made me feel worse, and so finally I was referred to a psychologist who prescribed narcosis (i.e. being sedated and put to sleep) which lasted three days. This failed to help, and so the psychologist suggested giving me a course of ECT. I was very frightened, really desperate, I felt as though I was cracking-up. It wasn't any wonder that my marriage split up. I even attempted suicide.*

*I just felt like I wanted to shut the door and be on my own, and yet I didn't want to be on my own, it was most peculiar.*

### I disliked myself

*I just felt a mess pre-menstrually. An absolute mess. I really didn't like myself at all. The thing was that in my teens I could cope with it, because it was*

*Despite the fact that most of the patients who volunteered to tell their story in the book didn't object to my using their actual names, I felt it would be more appropriate to change their names and let them remain anonymous.

*every few months and only for a day or two before my period. I was slimmer then and I had long blonde hair. As I got older and had Emma I just felt like a slob because everything had gone, everything had dropped, my skin was really terrible and itchy and my hair was greasy.*

### Relationships

*Steve and I had been married for ten years before he started retaliating. So he'd put up with me for a long time. He'd put up with a lot. I've thrown things down the stairs at him and even hit him right across the face in front of our daughter. He's 5 ft 10 ins (1 m 75 cm) and quite reserved and easy-going usually.*

*I can remember a day when he happened to mention the curtains I'd just hand-sewn were not wide enough. I flew into a rage and kicked him, then flew upstairs and cried. When I came down we started arguing and fighting over something else. That's when he started hitting back.*

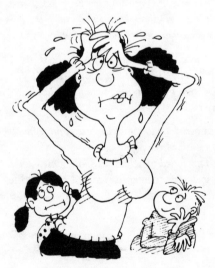

### My terrified little daughter

*Emma was a wonderful, active child and began talking by eight months. By twelve months she would answer back and be deliberately defiant. I could only put up with her for so long pre-menstrually and then I'd hit her. I knew I shouldn't have done that. I realize it now because she was only twelve months old. She's been smacked much more than she should have been.*

*She was growing up to be a frightened little girl. She just didn't know which way her mummy was going to be. She was very frightened of me, so much so, she didn't want to be left alone in the house with me, especially when I was pre-menstrual. That is a dreadful way for a child to be.*

### Hormone treatment

*After my overdose my doctor decided to try me on a hormone treatment. Shortly after I started on hormones I developed very severe breast tenderness. My breasts literally stood out and they were so sore and uncomfortable. I kept taking them for two months but the problem just intensified. I ended up taking pain killers every day to try to ease the pain.*

*I decided to stop taking the hormone treatment but that was easier said than done. I had awful withdrawal symptoms even though I came off them gradually. First I took two per day, then one, then every other day. The symptoms were so awful and, Oh my head! I've never known anything like it. I couldn't bear to put a foot down in front of me. The food cravings I had were unbelievable. I vowed I would never take another tablet for the rest of my life.*

### Relief at last

*I read about the Women's Nutritional Advisory Service in the local newspaper. I was at my wits' end at the time at the thought of spending another weekend in bed with terrible sweats and shakes. I felt like it was the last resort before I accepted the ECT. Fortunately, they managed to sort me out in the first five days, it was unbelievable!'*

Pauline suffered very severely with PMT, to the point where she was at times a danger to herself and certainly a liability to her family. Her whole life revolved around her pre-menstrual symptoms. She was, sadly, unable to lead a normal life and on the point of having psychiatric treatment, ECT, when she contacted us. (ECT, electroconvulsive therapy, electric shock treatment, kills brain cells and these do not regenerate.)

The chart from her first questionnaire has been copied above. This she completed when she first contacted us. You will notice that quite a few symptoms in each category were severe pre-menstrually. She was, in fact, suffering with all four categories of PMT listed. However, most of the symptoms in PMT A, the first category, were so severe that they were still present the week after her period. We soon discovered that this was largely due to her nutritional state and her diet. I will

# PRE-MENSTRUAL SYNDROME QUESTIONNAIRE

Name: __Pauline Solent__     Age: __35__     Height: __5′ 5″__     Weight: __9st 10lb__

MARITAL STATUS:     Single _____     Married __✓__     Divorced _____     Widowed _____
(Please tick where applicable)

PRESENT CONTRACEPTION:     None __✓__     Pill _____     I.U.D. _____     Other _____

    Your periods come every __31–33__ days     Your periods last __7__ days

    Your periods are:   Light _____     Moderate _____     Heavy __✓__

    Number of Pregnancies: __1__     Number of Miscarriages: _____

Birth weight of children   1st Child __6lb 4oz__   2nd Child _____   3rd Child _____   4th Child _____

| SYMPTOMS | WEEK AFTER PERIOD (Fill in 3 days after period) | | | | WEEK BEFORE PERIOD (Fill in 2-3 days before period) | | | |
|---|---|---|---|---|---|---|---|---|
| | None | Mild | Moderate | Severe | None | Mild | Moderate | Severe |
| **PMT - A** | | | | | | | | |
| Nervous Tension | | | | ✓ | | | | ✓ |
| Mood Swings | ✓ | | | | | | | ✓ |
| Irritability | | | ✓ | | | | | ✓ |
| Anxiety | | | ✓ | | | | | ✓ |
| **PMT - H** | | | | | | | | |
| Weight gain | ✓ | | | | ✓ | | | |
| Swelling of Extremities | ✓ | | | | ✓ | | | |
| Breast Tenderness | ✓ | | | | | | | |
| Abdominal Bloating | ✓ | | | | | | | |
| **PMT - C** | | | | | | | | |
| Headache | | | ✓ | | | | | ✓ |
| Craving for Sweets | ✓ | | | | | | | ✓ |
| Increased Appetite | ✓ | | | | | ✓ | | |
| Heart Pounding | ✓ | | | | | | | |
| Fatigue | | | ✓ | | | | | ✓ |
| Dizziness or Fainting | | | ✓ | | | | | ✓ |
| **PMT - D** | | | | | | | | |
| Depression | | | | ✓ | | | | |
| Forgetfulness | ✓ | | | | | | | |
| Crying | | | ✓ | | | | | |
| Confusion | ✓ | | | | | | | |
| Insomnia | | | | ✓ | | | | |
| **OTHER SYMPTOMS** | | | | | | | | |
| Loss of Sexual Interest | | | | ✓ | | | | ✓ |
| Disorientation | ✓ | | | | ✓ | | | |
| Clumsiness | ✓ | | | | | | | ✓ |
| Tremors/Shakes | ✓ | | | | | | | ✓ |
| Thoughts of Suicide | | ✓ | | | | | | ✓ |
| Agoraphobia | | | ✓ | | | | | ✓ |
| Increased Physical Activity | ✓ | | | | ✓ | | | |
| Heavy/Aching Legs | ✓ | | | | ✓ | | | |
| Generalized Aches | ✓ | | | | | | | ✓ |
| Bad Breath | ✓ | | | | ✓ | | | |
| Sensitivity to Music/Light | ✓ | | | | | | | ✓ |
| Excessive Thirst | ✓ | | | | | | | ✓ |

## FOLLOW UP
## PRE-MENSTRUAL SYNDROME QUESTIONNAIRE

Name: _Pauline Solent_    Age: _35_    Height: _5' 5"_    Weight: _9st 2lb_

MARITAL STATUS:    Single_____    Married___✓___    Divorced_____    Widowed_____
(Please tick where applicable)

PRESENT CONTRACEPTION:    None___✓___    Pill_____    I.U.D._____    Other_____

   Your periods come every _31–33_ days    Your periods last _5–7_ days

   Your periods are:    Light_____    Moderate___✓___    Heavy_____

| SYMPTOMS | WEEK AFTER PERIOD (Fill in 3 days after period) | | | | WEEK BEFORE PERIOD (Fill in 2-3 days before period) | | | |
|---|---|---|---|---|---|---|---|---|
| | None | Mild | Moderate | Severe | None | Mild | Moderate | Severe |
| **PMT - A** | | | | | | | | |
| Nervous Tension | ✓ | | | | ✓ | | | |
| Mood Swings | ✓ | | | | ✓ | | | |
| Irritability | ✓ | | | | ✓ | | | |
| Anxiety | ✓ | | | | ✓ | | | |
| **PMT - H** | | | | | | | | |
| Weight gain | ✓ | | | | ✓ | | | |
| Swelling of Extremities | ✓ | | | | ✓ | | | |
| Breast Tenderness | ✓ | | | | ✓ | | | |
| Abdominal Bloating | ✓ | | | | ✓ | | | |
| **PMT - C** | | | | | | | | |
| Headache | ✓ | | | | ✓ | | | |
| Craving for Sweets | ✓ | | | | ✓ | | | |
| Increased Appetite | ✓ | | | | ✓ | | | |
| Heart Pounding | ✓ | | | | ✓ | | | |
| Fatigue | ✓ | | | | ✓ | | | |
| Dizziness or Fainting | ✓ | | | | ✓ | | | |
| **PMT - D** | | | | | | | | |
| Depression | ✓ | | | | ✓ | | | |
| Forgetfulness | ✓ | | | | ✓ | | | |
| Crying | ✓ | | | | ✓ | | | |
| Confusion | ✓ | | | | ✓ | | | |
| Insomnia | ✓ | | | | ✓ | | | |
| **OTHER SYMPTOMS** | | | | | | | | |
| Loss of Sexual Interest | ✓ | | | | ✓ | | | |
| Disorientation | ✓ | | | | ✓ | | | |
| Clumsiness | ✓ | | | | ✓ | | | |
| Tremors/Shakes | ✓ | | | | ✓ | | | |
| Thoughts of Suicide | ✓ | | | | ✓ | | | |
| Agoraphobia | ✓ | | | | ✓ | | | |
| Increased Physical Activity | ✓ | | | | ✓ | | | |
| Heavy/Aching Legs | ✓ | | | | ✓ | | | |
| Generalized Aches | ✓ | | | | ✓ | | | |
| Bad Breath | ✓ | | | | ✓ | | | |
| Sensitivity to Music/Light | ✓ | | | | ✓ | | | |
| Excessive Thirst | ✓ | | | | ✓ | | | |

explain this more fully in the Diet section on page 137. She admits herself that she responded exceedingly quickly to a change in diet and nutritional supplements of vitamins and minerals.

### Previous diet

'I used to drink nine or 10 cups of tea per day and I used a lot of salt both in my cooking and at the table. I ate lots of convenience foods like pre-packed pies and tinned foods and I ate a fair amount of cheese, milk and wholemeal (wholewheat) bread. Also, I could easily eat four or five biscuits a day.

### New diet

I think the diet suggested by the Women's Nutritional Advisory Service is wonderful. I found it a little difficult at first but I think that's because my head was so peculiar pre-menstrually that I couldn't take it all in.

When the programme arrived I drove to my mum's and we sat down together and read through it so that we understood it fully. She then came with me to the supermarket and I bought lots of leeks, fresh vegetables and fruit, salad and fish. I had to cut out wholewheat and all foods containing yeast. I was given lists of foods to avoid and lists of food to concentrate on. I eat loads of fresh food now and feel wonderful. My friends all know I'm on a special diet. It's become a way of life now.'

Pauline's follow-up questionnaire after six months looks dramatically different. All her pre-menstrual symptoms are gone completely.

### End result

'I don't have any symptoms any more. My life has changed dramatically. I feel much more at ease and I never shout, unless I am very angry.

My agoraphobia has gone completely. I can go out with confidence and I feel great in myself. I can do all the things I couldn't do before. I can go anywhere.

Steve and I get on really well now, so much so we are even planning to have another baby, which I could never have coped with before. I had no intention of having any more children, in fact I'd given away all the baby equipment. I am truly delighted with the results of my programme. My husband thinks it's wonderful too.'

From a letter Pauline sent at the end of her programme you can tell she is now coping with life and feels normal again.

*Dear Maryon,*

*I am very fit now and I have just spent a hectic week in London with my six-year-old daughter – who is a handful. I feel marvellous. She's been better as I have practically put her on my diet (except she does have some sweets), and she watches my diet.*

*Thanks again for giving me my life back after 20 years.*

*Yours ever so grateful*
*Pauline Solent*

## " Ruth's Story "

Ruth was another victim of violent and aggressive feelings which she acted on pre-menstrually. Classically, she didn't experience any of these feelings once her period arrived.

Ruth is a 39-year-old who is a housewife and a mother of two children. Her PMT began after the birth of her first baby, although she feels it may have been simmering beforehand.

*'PMT totally changed my character when I had it, and I had it for half my life. It began two weeks before my period, sometimes more. It would disappear on the first day of my period and I immediately felt a sense of relief. Then a week after my period it began to build up again.*

*I became very irritable, very tired, snappy and aggressive, which is not a bit what I'm like normally. I would shout at my husband, literally scream at him. I think I still have sore throats as a result. I used to go to my room and have a screaming fit to keep it to myself. But people would aggravate me easily. Obviously when you have small children they tend to get on your nerves when you are tired. I felt like a lump of lead at the time and I know I had very little patience with my older daughter who was my only child when it was at its worst. She suffered, I'm sure. I would scream at her and hit her at times which was very upsetting for me afterwards because I know a child of seven couldn't possibly understand.*

### I vowed it wouldn't happen next month

*Although my husband was understanding and sympathetic, it's very difficult to have a normal relationship with someone when they are aggressive and not well.*

37

There is no doubt about the fact that the presence of PMT symptoms placed a strain on our marriage.

I suppose everybody has irritating habits and normally I would just take them in my stride. But at PMT times my husband would aggravate me to the point where I'd scream at him. Unfortunately it was over stupid, insignificant things.

Very often I'd take it out on the children instead of my husband. This was because I knew he had such high standards of self-discipline and I think he felt that I ought to have been able to do something about my own behaviour. I always vowed that next month I was jolly well going to, it was mind over matter etc., but it never seemed to work.

### I hated myself

When pre-menstrual I felt I was awful, I really hated myself. When I started hitting my daughter, I felt like I had really failed myself. I felt like a worm. Really dreadful. I cannot explain how I felt. My usual philosophy is that if children are treated right they respond and they are not naughty. I tried to explain to my doctor but he didn't understand. I remember shouting at him "you don't understand" but he just threw his hands up in horror and walked out of the surgery.

### My daughter locked herself away from me

I think my daughter was quite frightened of me actually. I am normally placid but of course I wasn't, as my symptoms were occurring more often than not when I was at my worst.

The problem would usually begin over a trivial matter which now I would brush aside or cope with calmly. Then I would just feel so tight inside and of course, it would then become a big thing. Of course with children if you build it up they build it up also, and it all gets out of hand. I would sometimes grip her and shake her, poor girl. It was a dreadful way to treat a child. She would often go off and lock herself in her bedroom because she was afraid of me.

I never did her any bad damage, but it was awful to me as I would never normally strike a child. I don't agree with bashing children when they are naughty, particularly as she probably wasn't even that naughty. It just got out of hand.

### Previous treatments

The first time I went to the doctor about my PMT, and I have been to several doctors about it over the years, it was thought a good idea for me to take *the Pill to remove the "tension" beforehand. This was after the birth of my first child, about 14 years ago. The Pill caused me awful headaches and I had to come off it.*

*I realized I couldn't continue to suffer, by which time my original doctor had left the practice. The new doctor prescribed vitamin B6. He wanted to try the natural approach first before prescribing progesterone. Although I thought that the vitamin B6 was helping at first, it didn't make the slightest difference to my symptoms.*

*I then read that evening primrose oil might help, so I bought some. I have still got the remains of the bottle, unfortunately. It didn't help at all.*

*I saw a specialist who examined me thoroughly and could find nothing physically wrong. He said it was a hormonal imbalance and prescribed hormone treatment. I was never very happy about taking hormones, I would rather have taken more natural things. They did help my symptoms though, to the point where I could function to some degree. But PMT reared its ugly head again. It would pop up now and then. It was not fully quashed. Life wasn't what I would describe as being bearable, but it was more under control than before.*

*My husband then read an article in the newspaper about the nutritional programme for PMT being so successful and suggested I follow that up.'*

Ruth struggled for 14 years with her symptoms. Again, it affected a large portion of her life. She admits her family suffered a great deal because of her behaviour pre-menstrually. And in common with all the other sufferers mentioned, she was unable to control herself. When her period began all her symptoms went.

She suffered severely with three categories of PMT: PMT A, the nervous and uptight symptoms, PMT C, craving for sweet foods etc., and PMT D, particularly depression, confusion and forgetfulness. She had tried many treatments before to help ease her symptoms, but she was unable to control the situation. Long-term hormone treatment did help to ease things a bit, but she was unhappy taking them.

Her first chart is on page 40.

### Diet helped

*'I really had no idea that diet was an important factor in controlling PMT. I thought it was a question of hormone balance being wrong. And the only way to put it right was to put in more hormones, the right kind of hormones, rather than eat different things.*

# PRE-MENSTRUAL SYNDROME QUESTIONNAIRE

Name: __Ruth Sears__          Age: __39__     Height: __5' 11"__     Weight: __12st__

MARITAL STATUS:     Single _____     Married ___✓___     Divorced _____     Widowed _____
(Please tick where applicable)

PRESENT CONTRACEPTION:     None _____     Pill _____     I.U.D. __✓__     Other _____

    Your periods come every __28__ days          Your periods last ___5___ days

    Your periods are: Light _____     Moderate __✓__     Heavy _____

    Number of Pregnancies: ___3___     Number of Miscarriages: ___1___

Birth weight of children:  1st Child __7lb 15oz__  2nd Child __8lb 10oz__  3rd Child _____  4th Child _____

| SYMPTOMS | WEEK AFTER PERIOD (Fill in 3 days after period) | | | | WEEK BEFORE PERIOD (Fill in 2-3 days before period) | | | |
|---|---|---|---|---|---|---|---|---|
| | None | Mild | Moderate | Severe | None | Mild | Moderate | Severe |
| **PMT - A** | | | | | | | | |
| Nervous Tension | ✓ | | | | | | | ✓ |
| Mood Swings | ✓ | | | | | | | ✓ |
| Irritability | ✓ | | | | | | | ✓ |
| Anxiety | ✓ | | | | | | ✓ | |
| **PMT - H** | | | | | | | | |
| Weight gain | ✓ | | | | | | ✓ | |
| Swelling of Extremities | ✓ | | | | ✓ | | | |
| Breast Tenderness | ✓ | | | | ✓ | | | |
| Abdominal Bloating | ✓ | | | | | | ✓ | |
| **PMT - C** | | | | | | | | |
| Headache | ✓ | | | | ✓ | | | |
| Craving for Sweets | ✓ | | | | | | | ✓ |
| Increased Appetite | ✓ | | | | | | | ✓ |
| Heart Pounding | ✓ | | | | ✓ | | | |
| Fatigue | ✓ | | | | | | | ✓ |
| Dizziness or Fainting | ✓ | | | | ✓ | | | |
| **PMT - D** | | | | | | | | |
| Depression | ✓ | | | | | | | ✓ |
| Forgetfulness | ✓ | | | | | | | ✓ |
| Crying | ✓ | | | | ✓ | | | |
| Confusion | ✓ | | | | | | | ✓ |
| Insomnia | ✓ | | | | ✓ | | | |
| **OTHER SYMPTOMS** | | | | | | | | |
| Loss of Sexual Interest | ✓ | | | | | | | ✓ |
| Disorientation | ✓ | | | | | | ✓ | |
| Clumsiness | ✓ | | | | | | ✓ | |
| Tremors/Shakes | ✓ | | | | ✓ | | | |
| Thoughts of Suicide | ✓ | | | | ✓ | | | |
| Agoraphobia | ✓ | | | | ✓ | | | |
| Increased Physical Activity | ✓ | | | | ✓ | | | |
| Heavy/Aching Legs | ✓ | | | | ✓ | | | |
| Generalized Aches | ✓ | | | | ✓ | | | |
| Bad Breath | ✓ | | | | ✓ | | | |
| Sensitivity to Music/Light | ✓ | | | | ✓ | | | |
| Excessive Thirst | ✓ | | | | ✓ | | | |

I used to drink quite a bit of coffee, add lots of salt to my food, and I had a lot of sugary foods. I used to try to eat a high fibre and low fat diet because I was always trying to get my weight down. I did have a weakness for chocolates and biscuits, in fact I used to crave them especially pre-menstrually.

I read an article in the newspaper about the Women's Nutritional Advisory Service dietary recommendations, so I was semi-prepared when I received my programme. Being asked to cut out grains shocked me a bit. It was the most complicated part of the diet, I found, as so many things contain wheat.

I did stick to the diet to the letter for the first three months. I even had a special meal prepared when we attended a formal dinner. No one asked why, and I didn't want to mention the reason. They were all very discreet about it. It didn't cause a problem.

My symptoms completely vanished on the programme. It was absolute magic. Even my long-standing problem of thrush cleared up when I was avoiding wheat and foods containing yeast.

I am back on all the usual foods now. I no longer have the intense sweet cravings and I feel I know where to draw the line. I still take Optivite, a vitamin supplement which I think is marvellous, and my symptoms haven't returned.

I'm delighted to say that my life has been transformed since starting on the programme. I followed the suggested diet very closely for six months and took the recommended vitamin and mineral supplements. In fact, I still take the supplements but have been able to moderate my diet. It seems amazing to me that such strong, violent symptoms could be controlled by changing my diet and taking some vitamin pills.'

Her follow-up questionnaire reflects her progress. Most symptoms are completely under control. Just a bit of mild breast tenderness pre-menstrually remains.

### End result

'Since undertaking the nutritional programme to overcome my PMT, I can honestly say my symptoms have disappeared. I think they have really vanished, like absolute magic. I am overwhelmed by it. My life is now back to normal. There is no comparison in me now. I am a completely different woman. Back to what I was before.'

Ruth's letter to me at the end of her programme was interesting as she points out that it is sometimes genuinely difficult to come off treatment – even if it isn't really

# FOLLOW UP
## PRE-MENSTRUAL SYNDROME QUESTIONNAIRE

Name: _Ruth Sears_    Age: _39_    Height: _5' 11"_    Weight: _12st_

MARITAL STATUS:    Single _____    Married _✓_    Divorced _____    Widowed _____
(Please tick where applicable)

PRESENT CONTRACEPTION:    None _____    Pill _____    I.U.D. _✓_    Other _____

     Your periods come every _28_ days      Your periods last _5_ days

     Your periods are:   Light _____    Moderate _✓_    Heavy _____

| SYMPTOMS | WEEK AFTER PERIOD (Fill in 3 days after period) | | | | WEEK BEFORE PERIOD (Fill in 2-3 days before period) | | | |
|---|---|---|---|---|---|---|---|---|
| | None | Mild | Moderate | Severe | None | Mild | Moderate | Severe |
| **PMT - A** | | | | | | | | |
| Nervous Tension | ✓ | | | | ✓ | | | |
| Mood Swings | ✓ | | | | ✓ | | | |
| Irritability | ✓ | | | | ✓ | | | |
| Anxiety | ✓ | | | | ✓ | | | |
| **PMT - H** | | | | | | | | |
| Weight gain | ✓ | | | | ✓ | | | |
| Swelling of Extremities | ✓ | | | | ✓ | | | |
| Breast Tenderness | ✓ | | | | | | ✓ | |
| Abdominal Bloating | | ✓ | | | ✓ | | | |
| **PMT - C** | | | | | | | | |
| Headache | ✓ | | | | ✓ | | | |
| Craving for Sweets | ✓ | | | | ✓ | | | |
| Increased Appetite | ✓ | | | | ✓ | | | |
| Heart Pounding | ✓ | | | | ✓ | | | |
| Fatigue | ✓ | ✓ | | | ✓ | | | |
| Dizziness or Fainting | ✓ | | | | ✓ | | | |
| **PMT - D** | | | | | | | | |
| Depression | ✓ | | | | ✓ | | | |
| Forgetfulness | ✓ | | | | ✓ | | | |
| Crying | ✓ | | | | ✓ | | | |
| Confusion | ✓ | | | | ✓ | | | |
| Insomnia | ✓ | | | | ✓ | | | |
| **OTHER SYMPTOMS** | | | | | | | | |
| Loss of Sexual Interest | ✓ | | | | ✓ | | | |
| Disorientation | ✓ | | | | ✓ | | | |
| Clumsiness | ✓ | | | | ✓ | | | |
| Tremors/Shakes | ✓ | | | | ✓ | | | |
| Thoughts of Suicide | ✓ | | | | ✓ | | | |
| Agoraphobia | ✓ | | | | ✓ | | | |
| Increased Physical Activity | ✓ | | | | ✓ | | | |
| Heavy/Aching Legs | ✓ | | | | ✓ | | | |
| Generalized Aches | ✓ | | | | ✓ | | | |
| Bad Breath | ✓ | | | | ✓ | | | |
| Sensitivity to Music/Light | ✓ | | | | ✓ | | | |
| Excessive Thirst | ✓ | | | | ✓ | | | |

working. Trying a new approach does often involve courage, especially when so many other treatments have failed previously.

*Dear Maryon,*

*I am enclosing my follow-up questionnaire and must take the opportunity to tell you how absolutely the course has changed my life. I couldn't have believed that just vitamins, minerals and a change of diet could have such a dramatic impact.*

*Having had quite severe symptoms it was an act of courage and determination to break off the progesterone treatment and step into the blue on your programme. I'm glad I did.*

*Ruth Sears*

Here is another example of how PMT A symptoms affected the life of a young single woman, who was also diagnosed as having irritable bowel syndrome.

Nadine is a 25-year-old single woman who works as an advertising executive. She has been suffering with PMT since she was 15 years of age and feels that her life has been pretty disrupted as a result.

## " Nadine's Story "

'I felt trapped like a victim, trapped in the philosophy of being a woman and stuck with it. I was very fed up with the suffering every month, it was like being in a biological prison. I was very frightened.

PMT just meant misery to me, it made my life difficult and extremely unpleasant. That's the best way I can explain it. The fact that I had no idea what it was, made matters worse. From the age of 15 I was extremely unpleasant premenstrually, to my mother in particular. I would start shouting at her. I was very aggressive and argumentative before my period. Unfortunately, I wasn't aware of the pattern at the time.

My social life was affected by my symptoms and at work I just got a reputation for being an extremely rude person. In fact, previously at college I had been nicknamed "The Misery".

I used to take my frustrations out on my boyfriend. I'd lash out at him with my fists, then I would throw things around the room. That was the worst thing, *feeling so aggressive and throwing things around. He would try to calm me down by cuddling me. He knew if he rode the storm that I would calm down eventually when my period came.*

*My tummy problems were so severe I was diagnosed by my doctor as having irritable bowel syndrome, caused by stress. I felt that that was a very convenient diagnosis to make when he didn't really know what the problem was and he wanted to get rid of me. "Tell them it's stress and they'll go away."*

*I felt pretty awful. I tried to help myself by taking some vitamin B6, then I tried evening primrose oil and zinc, and finally my doctor prescribed progesterone suppositories. None of the treatments were successful, though.*

*It wasn't until I read articles in magazines about the work that the Women's Nutritional Advisory Service was doing that I came to realize that I was suffering from PMT. Up until then I was just aware that my symptoms were getting worse and worse and I didn't know what to do about them.'*

Nadine is a young, single woman who has not had any children. Nevertheless, at the time she came to us she had been suffering with PMT symptoms for some ten years. Her main problem areas were the tension and anxiety symptoms, and the swelling and bloating symptoms, as you can see from her chart.

Understandably, she was frightened about the effect that her ever-recurring symptoms had on her body and on her life. All areas of her life were disrupted because of her symptoms, and despite trying a series of treatments, both independently, and through her doctor, her symptoms showed no sign of easing off. The thought of going through her whole life suffering in this manner had been pretty uncomfortable to Nadine.

### Diet

*'My previous diet obviously wasn't right, in retrospect. I had a very bad stomach problem, in fact I was diagnosed as having irritable bowel disease. I had loads of unpleasant tests and was told that the condition was due to stress.*

*I used to get terrible diarrhoea and pain cramps in my tummy. The doctors told me to eat more bran, which I have since found out aggravates the condition.*

*I didn't know that diet could play such an important role. I did wonder sometimes though. I did a degree in Food Science and there was a small amount of information on the effects that diet could have on the body. Although I had my suspicions, I didn't know how to go about finding out more. I did try looking for*

# PRE-MENSTRUAL SYNDROME QUESTIONNAIRE

Name: _Nadine Morris_          Age: _25_          Height: _5' 2"_          Weight: _10st 4lb_

MARITAL STATUS:          Single __✓__          Married _____          Divorced _____          Widowed _____
(Please tick where applicable)

PRESENT CONTRACEPTION:          None _____          Pill _____          I.U.D. _____          Other __✓__

Your periods come every _27–35_ days          Your periods last _4–5_ days

Your periods are:   Light _____          Moderate __✓__          Heavy _____

Number of Pregnancies: _1_          Number of Miscarriages: _1_

Birth weight of children:   1st Child _____   2nd Child _____   3rd Child _____   4th Child _____

| SYMPTOMS | WEEK AFTER PERIOD (Fill in 3 days after period) | | | | WEEK BEFORE PERIOD (Fill in 2-3 days before period) | | | |
|---|---|---|---|---|---|---|---|---|
| | None | Mild | Moderate | Severe | None | Mild | Moderate | Severe |
| **PMT - A** | | | | | | | | |
| Nervous Tension | ✓ | | | | | | | ✓ |
| Mood Swings | ✓ | | | | | | | ✓ |
| Irritability | ✓ | | | | | | | ✓ |
| Anxiety | | ✓ | | | | | | ✓ |
| **PMT - H** | | | | | | | | |
| Weight gain | ✓ | | | | | | ✓ | |
| Swelling of Extremities | ✓ | | | | ✓ | | | |
| Breast Tenderness | ✓ | | | | | | ✓ | |
| Abdominal Bloating | | ✓ | | | | | | ✓ |
| **PMT - C** | | | | | | | | |
| Headache | ✓ | | | | ✓ | | | |
| Craving for Sweets | ✓ | | | | | ✓ | | |
| Increased Appetite | ✓ | | | | | ✓ | | |
| Heart Pounding | ✓ | | | | ✓ | | | |
| Fatigue | ✓ | | | | ✓ | | | |
| Dizziness or Fainting | ✓ | | | | ✓ | | | |
| **PMT - D** | | | | | | | | |
| Depression | ✓ | | | | ✓ | | | |
| Forgetfulness | ✓ | | | | ✓ | | | |
| Crying | ✓ | | | | | ✓ | | |
| Confusion | ✓ | | | | ✓ | | | |
| Insomnia | ✓ | | | | ✓ | | | |
| **OTHER SYMPTOMS** | | | | | | | | |
| Loss of Sexual Interest | ✓ | | | | ✓ | | | |
| Disorientation | ✓ | | | | ✓ | | | |
| Clumsiness | | ✓ | | | | | | ✓ |
| Tremors/Shakes | ✓ | | | | ✓ | | | |
| Thoughts of Suicide | ✓ | | | | ✓ | | | |
| Agoraphobia | | | | | | | | |
| Increased Physical Activity | | ✓ | | | ✓ | | | |
| Heavy/Aching Legs | ✓ | | | | ✓ | | | |
| Generalized Aches | ✓ | | | | ✓ | | | |
| Bad Breath | ✓ | | | | ✓ | | | |
| Sensitivity to Music/Light | ✓ | | | | ✓ | | | |
| Excessive Thirst | ✓ | | | | | | | ✓ |

*papers but I didn't really find many and I didn't find anything to connect diet to PMT or my irritable bowel problem.*

*I used to eat up to four slices of wholemeal (wholewheat) bread per day and have a bowl of bran. I also drank about five cups of tea per day, an extra $^3/_4$ of a pint (450 ml) of milk per day, and other dairy foods.*

*On my programme I was asked to cut out grains, dairy products, yeast-based foods, tea and foods containing sugar. I stuck to the diet to the letter. It was inconvenient at first because it was so different. It took me a week or two to adapt and then it became easier.*

*Miraculously, soon after I began the diet my tummy problems just cleared up. I now know through trial and error that wheat and dairy products are irritants and will cause my diarrhoea to return.*

*I have relaxed my diet now that I am so much better. I am still fairly strict with myself most of the time. I can get away with drinking alcohol occasionally and sometimes I do eat processed foods or crisps.*

### End result

*Now that I have followed the nutritional programme, I have learned so much. My body has recovered from all the ailments, including my PMT and the irritable bowel syndrome. All the remaining traces of agoraphobia which I had previously suffered from in my late teens and early twenties have disappeared, and my skin condition has improved. My energy has just soared and I feel that I have come from being a poorly, lethargic person suddenly to someone who is healthy all the time. I am my usual bouncy self once again and I get on well with people. I don't experience the miseries any more, I am relieved to say.*

*I honestly feel that the Women's Nutritional Advisory Service has transformed my life. I used to think life was terrible. Now I find life pleasurable. I feel healthier than I have ever done, at least since I was a child. I can't thank them enough.'*

Nadine had no symptoms whatsoever left at the end of her six-month programme, as you can see from her chart.

An extract from a letter explains how Nadine felt about her programme.

*'I wanted to make some additional comments regarding the programme, apart from those in the accompanying questionnaire.*

## FOLLOW UP
## PRE-MENSTRUAL SYNDROME QUESTIONNAIRE

Name: __Nadine Morris__  Age: __25__  Height: __5' 2"__  Weight: __9st 9lb__

MARITAL STATUS:  Single __✓__  Married_____  Divorced_____  Widowed_____
(Please tick where applicable)

PRESENT CONTRACEPTION:  None_____  Pill_____  I.U.D. _____  Other __✓__

Your periods come every __28–35__ days  Your periods last __4–5__ days

Your periods are:  Light_____  Moderate __✓__  Heavy_____

| SYMPTOMS | WEEK AFTER PERIOD (Fill in 3 days after period) | | | | WEEK BEFORE PERIOD (Fill in 2-3 days before period) | | | |
|---|---|---|---|---|---|---|---|---|
| | None | Mild | Moderate | Severe | None | Mild | Moderate | Severe |
| **PMT - A** | | | | | | | | |
| Nervous Tension | ✓ | | | | ✓ | | | |
| Mood Swings | ✓ | | | | ✓ | | | |
| Irritability | ✓ | | | | ✓ | | | |
| Anxiety | ✓ | | | | ✓ | | | |
| **PMT - H** | | | | | | | | |
| Weight gain | ✓ | | | | ✓ | | | |
| Swelling of Extremities | ✓ | | | | ✓ | | | |
| Breast Tenderness | ✓ | | | | ✓ | | | |
| Abdominal Bloating | ✓ | | | | ✓ | | | |
| **PMT - C** | | | | | | | | |
| Headache | ✓ | | | | ✓ | | | |
| Craving for Sweets | ✓ | | | | ✓ | | | |
| Increased Appetite | ✓ | | | | ✓ | | | |
| Heart Pounding | ✓ | | | | ✓ | | | |
| Fatigue | ✓ | | | | ✓ | | | |
| Dizziness or Fainting | ✓ | | | | ✓ | | | |
| **PMT - D** | | | | | | | | |
| Depression | ✓ | | | | ✓ | | | |
| Forgetfulness | ✓ | | | | ✓ | | | |
| Crying | ✓ | | | | ✓ | | | |
| Confusion | ✓ | | | | ✓ | | | |
| Insomnia | ✓ | | | | ✓ | | | |
| **OTHER SYMPTOMS** | | | | | | | | |
| Loss of Sexual Interest | ✓ | | | | ✓ | | | |
| Disorientation | ✓ | | | | ✓ | | | |
| Clumsiness | ✓ | | | | ✓ | | | |
| Tremors/Shakes | ✓ | | | | ✓ | | | |
| Thoughts of Suicide | ✓ | | | | ✓ | | | |
| Agoraphobia | ✓ | | | | ✓ | | | |
| Increased Physical Activity | ✓ | | | | ✓ | | | |
| Heavy/Aching Legs | ✓ | | | | ✓ | | | |
| Generalized Aches | ✓ | | | | ✓ | | | |
| Bad Breath | ✓ | | | | ✓ | | | |
| Sensitivity to Music/Light | ✓ | | | | ✓ | | | |
| Excessive Thirst | ✓ | | | | ✓ | | | |

*First of all, I'd like to thank you for such detailed information and guidance in your letter of recommendations. The programme has made the biological and physiological aspects of womanhood a great deal easier to cope with. My periods are much less painful and lighter. The gruesome week before my period, which was always so unbearable, is now like the other two weeks. I no longer suffer from any breast tenderness, which used to be so severe, and no longer suffer with bloatedness. I no longer hate everything and everybody including myself, and I no longer feel violent or aggressive, which is a very great relief. I also don't wreck everything around me through clumsiness, as that's gone too.*

*All in all, the programme has transformed me and my life quite remarkably and I am grateful for the work you and your colleagues have done to enable me to live without dreading the onset of each period. More significantly, I feel that the diet and discovery of foods that I am allergic to has improved my whole life, not just my PMT.*

*For about seven years I have suffered with irritable bowel syndrome, more recently it became so bad that I was referred to a specialist who, after various unpleasant tests, pronounced it was caused by stress. Ironically most doctors have prescribed increased intake of wholewheat products and bran, no wonder I wasn't getting any better! Admittedly, when I am in a stressful situation my symptoms return, but they last only as long as the stress. Previously, the irritable bowel symptoms were with me constantly and just became unbearable when I was under stress.*

*I know this isn't entirely relevant to your work on PMT but at the same time many of my female contemporaries seem to suffer from irritable bowel syndrome too and I wonder how many woman are being inappropriately treated and dismissed with mutterings of ''it's psychosomatic''?*

*I hope my comments have been some help in your work to relieve the misery of PMT. I for one am a very grateful and satisfied customer!'*

*Yours sincerely*
*Nadine*

# 6

# BLOATING, WEIGHT GAIN AND BREAST TENDERNESS

## PMT H (HYDRATION)

PMT H sufferers complain of weight gain pre-menstrually. The hands and feet often swell so that rings and shoes become too tight. The face often becomes puffy and the waistline expands so that clothes feel too tight. The abdomen can become bloated and tender and the same applies to the breasts.

The manifestations of these symptoms are mostly physical, in that women report feeling very uncomfortable and often sore. Because of their increased size many women feel self-conscious and get very touchy and introverted. Surprisingly, most women who suffer from PMT H only gain up to 3–4 pounds (1–2 kg) pre-menstrually. Approximately 20 per cent seem to gain far more than this. I have personally seen women who gain up to 12 pounds (5.4 kg) before their periods. They literally change dress size and need to have two sets of underwear to cope with their increased breast size.

PMT H is similar to PMT A in that it is thought that oestrogen is too high and progesterone is too low. Although having said that, normal levels of oestrogen have been observed in some women with PMT H.

As I explained in PMT A, when oestrogen levels are too high, an excessive amount of brain chemicals is produced, including a chemical called serotonin. Too much serotonin causes the body to produce more of a hormone called aldosterone.

This hormone is produced by the adrenal glands, which are situated just above the kidneys. These glands control the kidneys' water and salt retention. Aldosterone, when balanced, is an essential hormone. But in excessive amounts it causes the body to retain water and salt, hence the bloating occurs.

In addition to these hormonal factors, intake of salt (sodium chloride) is also important. Some women will retain fluid, not just pre-menstrually, if their salt intake is too high. This effect can be aggravated by a high intake of sugar or of refined carbohydrate foods. When this is a problem a low salt diet, avoiding the use of salt in cooking, at the table and many salty foods, e.g. salty crisps, bacon, cheese, pickles, etc., needs to be followed. For some women careful adherence to such a diet may have a very beneficial effect.

However, some women who complain of pre-menstrual abdominal bloating and puffy fingers do not have an increase in body water and salt content. It may be that their perception of their body changes and they just 'feel' different.

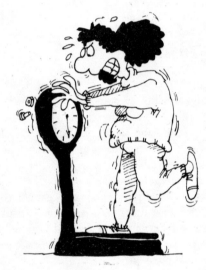

## THE DEGREE OF SUFFERING

In our study we found that 90.8 per cent of the women complained of abdominal bloating to some degree, (72 per cent severe to moderately).

Of the women studied 86.8 per cent had pre-menstrual breast tenderness (67 per cent severe to moderate sufferers).

Weight was gained by 84 per cent (52 per cent severe to moderately) and 54 per cent complained of swelling of the extremities (33 per cent severe to moderate).

| Degree of pre-menstrual breast tenderness suffered out of a sample of 1000 women | | | | |
| --- | --- | --- | --- | --- |
| Not Affected | Mild | Moderate | Severe | Total Affected |
| 13.2% | 19.9% | 31.6% | 35.3% - | 86.8% |

| Degree to which abdominal bloating affected a sample of 1000 women pre-menstrually | | | | |
| --- | --- | --- | --- | --- |
| Not Affected | Mild | Moderate | Severe | Total Affected |
| 9.2% | 18.5% | 39.3% | 33.0% - | 90.8% |

## WEIGHT LOSS

Whilst conducting our follow-up consultations during the programme, we began to notice that many overweight women who were previously unable to lose weight were enthusiastically reporting weight loss. This began occurring even after the first month, without even 'dieting' to lose weight. In fact, their intake of food during the programme was in many cases greater than usual.

Because of this somewhat unexpected outcome, we decided to monitor a group of 50 PMT sufferers who were also overweight, through the first three months of their programme. (Thirty-six of the women were at least 10 per cent overweight and 14 of them were obese, which means greater than 33 per cent above normal body weight.) The symptoms complained of most severely to begin with were weight gain, fatigue, abdominal bloating, craving for food, in particular sweet foods, and anxiety.

After three months on their programmes there was an 84 per cent reduction in severe symptoms.

51

The overweight group of 36 women lost an average of 7 pounds (3 kg) and the obese group of 14 women lost an average of 13 pounds (6 kg) in this three-month period.

We can't say precisely why this amount of weight loss had occurred, particularly when the women had previously found it difficult to lose weight. However, the common denominator seems to be that they were all on a healthy diet that had been balanced according to their individual needs. We therefore suspect that this must have had a positive effect on their metabolism with the result that they began to shed excess weight.

This is certainly an area we would like to research further. But in the meantime it's a gift horse that won't be looked in the mouth by PMT H sufferers.

## **((  Vivienne's Story  ))**

Vivienne is a 42-year-old woman from Sussex. She is married, has one child and works part time.

Vivienne's most severe problem was PMT H. The swelling and weight gain changed her physically to such a degree that she found it very hard to cope.

'After eating I would swell up within 20 minutes. The first thing I'd notice was an ache in my legs. It was like having a toothache or earache in your legs. It was very painful. I then got extreme fatigue which magnified my PMT symptoms. This was not helped by the fact that I looked seven or eight months pregnant. I even went to the Family Planning Clinic and was told by the doctor that there was no doubt that I was pregnant. After fully examining me she agreed I wasn't pregnant. I knew I couldn't be pregnant as I was on the Pill and having periods every month. The swelling was so severe it lasted all month. I didn't think it was period-related at first. However, when I began on the Nutritional Programme, I noticed my symptoms became pre-menstrual only. My breasts were so sore and swollen, though, it did make me wonder. I just didn't understand what was happening, that was the main thing.

I was put on diuretics which seemed to work well at first, but after a while they stopped working. I think my body must have got used to them.

I also suffered from severe pre-menstrual intolerance to situations. During that week all my worries were magnified out of proportion.

I was getting really desperate and happened to be recommended by a nurse to Dr Stewart. Fortunately, he's helped me to get to the bottom of the problem.

## A change of diet paid off

*I had no idea that diet was so relevant to my condition. I was asked to make considerable changes in my diet. Firstly, I had to leave out all the cereal-based foods, which was quite difficult. I also have a low-salt diet: that means not adding salt to food, besides avoiding food that has a high salt content. I have had to reduce sugar in my diet and cut down on foods containing animal fats. I now eat loads of vegetables and fruit.*

*I do find it difficult to stick to the diet, but I know it is worth it. For me, giving up foods was harder than giving up cigarettes.*

*When I do cheat on my diet I swell up within about 20 minutes, depending on what I've eaten and how much of it. Then at these times I really appreciate the importance of the diet. Basically, I think it's marvellous to be able to do without drugs and feel so much better, even if it is difficult to stick to.*

*I feel as if I have learned so much about diet now. I go and buy everything with no artificial colourings or preservatives. I avoid any junk food I can, as I know how complicated the problem can be if I put the wrong foods into my body.*

*My pre-menstrual time is very good now. I'm very pleased.'*

Vivienne had 'before' and 'after' laboratory tests during her treatment which showed that a change in diet was of great benefit.

## " Rebecca's Story "

Rebecca is a 38-year-old divorcee with two children who works as a teacher.

*'Looking back, I think my symptoms began increasing in severity after the birth of my children. Certainly, the last ten years have been the worst. I suffered for years before I even knew what I was suffering from. I'd never heard of "PMT". My doctor was unsympathetic, and so I thought it was just part of my make-up and therefore something I had to suffer.*

*My husband was very unsympathetic towards me during my pre-menstrual times. He couldn't believe I could be all right one minute and then suddenly have symptoms which involved him making adjustments. He really doubted that my symptoms actually existed. It caused a lot of misunderstandings and arguments. For example, I remember a time when I asked him to turn the record player down as it was giving me a headache, and he just grudgingly said, "Well, you were quite*

53

all right this morning". I just used to feel depressed, isolated and confused because I didn't really know why I was feeling so different pre-menstrually.

My symptoms would occur 10 to 12 days pre-menstrually. The most physically noticeable thing was that I'd gain four to five pounds (2–3 kg) in weight; my abdomen felt really bloated. I'd get cravings for food, in fact I just couldn't seem to get satisfied no matter what I ate. Apart from that I'd feel very irritable, exhausted and fairly afraid of my dizziness and fainting attacks, particularly when I went shopping or stood up for any length of time.

I looked terrible pre-menstrually, which didn't help. I had puffy eyes surrounded by dark shadows. Another thing was that I used to always feel cold, an inner cold. I would have to go to bed and crawl under the duvet with a hot-water bottle, but still wouldn't be able to overcome the cold; my teeth would still be chattering.

Life was really very difficult at the time and the stress of a broken marriage made things even worse. I found it difficult to work pre-menstrually as I couldn't concentrate. My head was so fuzzy and I couldn't formulate my ideas properly.

I had previously tried several different treatments for PMT, none of which were of any lasting value. I tried taking vitamin B6 on its own, but it didn't work. I also had some acupuncture and visited a medical herbalist. I put myself onto a course of Efamol evening primrose oil, but found that this only helped initially.

### Scatterbrain!

I was so forgetful. One day I put my handbag on the roof of the car whilst I loaded it and then I drove off without moving it! I can honestly say I felt terrible pre-menstrually. I didn't like myself at all.

### Wrecked marriage

My marriage broke down. I know that my PMT symptoms aggravated the situation. They caused a lot of misunderstandings. We had awful rows. He simply didn't believe my symptoms existed. I think he thought I'd made them up to suit myself and to inconvenience him. He had no understanding of the situation and I felt so isolated in it. I got very confused and tense as a result which aggravated my behaviour, so it was a vicious circle.'

Rebecca had severe symptoms in all four categories, pre-menstrually, whereas she had practically no symptoms at all at any other time of the month.

Rebecca also had 'before' and 'after' laboratory tests during her treatment which are detailed on page 135.

'When I heard about the nutritional approach to PMT, I decided to give it a go. I have been under Dr Stewart for over a year now. He has been measuring levels of vitamins and minerals in my body. I discovered I had an added complication of severe food allergies which we have also been working on, and a thyroid problem which is now being treated. My symptoms are down to a bearable two days per month now and I hope that I will be able to overcome them completely as time goes on.

Robert, with whom I now live, is very understanding and tolerant. Whenever I couldn't cope with a situation, he would just help me to do something. I'm sure it's due to his support that I have made it through.'

# 7

# SUGAR CRAVINGS, HEADACHES AND FATIGUE

## PMT C (CARBOHYDRATE CRAVING)

In this sub-group of PMT, one to two weeks before the period the appetite increases. Cravings for food begin, particularly for sweet foods and chocolate. Often stress intensifies the situation. Satisfying the cravings is a vicious circle. A typical example is as follows.

The day starts with either no breakfast or just a couple of cups of tea or coffee and a few cigarettes. This may stimulate the body's metabolism and one's energy for a short while, but the problems begin by mid-morning. By this time energy level tends to fall, and symptoms of nervousness, anxiety, palpitations, light headaches, hunger and cravings for food, particularly sweet foods, set in. Another cup of tea or coffee with sugar, or with a sugary or chocolate snack, may delay symptoms for a while but nothing short of a good wholesome meal will resolve these symptoms.

Some of these symptoms may be due to a fall in the level of sugar (glucose) in the blood – known as hypoglycaemia. As the brain and nervous system rely upon glucose for their source of energy, a fall in its level can cause a whole host of nervous system symptoms. The body compensates by producing adrenaline, which increases the level of glucose in the blood, but aggravates symptoms of anxiety, palpitations, sweating and shaking.

Such symptoms may be improved by the next meal. Often the mid-morning or mid-afternoon fatigue or sweet cravings are relieved by a wholesome lunch or supper.

Not all women will have such marked symptoms, nor indeed will there always

56

be marked swings in blood sugar levels. Often one just feels better if one eats three good meals a day, and has a regular, not too hectic lifestyle.

Headaches can also be caused by excessive intake of tea and coffee. Fatigue can be affected by the balance of minerals, such as iron and magnesium. Any women with persistent fatigue should certainly see her doctor for examination and appropriate blood tests, particularly to check for anaemia or reduced activity of the thyroid gland.

## GOOD FOOD REGULARLY, PLEASE!

So often the cravings for sweet foods, sugary snacks and chocolate are the result of an irregular and inadequate diet. Women with PMT C – carbohydrate cravings – may also experience headache, increased appetite, heart pounding, fatigue, and dizziness and fainting. These symptoms can be due to the swings in blood sugar levels and over-reliance on social stimulants: caffeine from tea, coffee, cola, chocolate, alcohol, cigarettes and even marijuana. Three good, regular meals, cutting down on sugar and social stimulants are all essential to treat PMT C.

## THE DEGREE OF SUFFERING

In our study we found that **77 per cent** of the women were suffering with cravings for sweet food, just over 60 per cent severe to moderately. There were **93 per cent** who reported suffering with fatigue pre-menstrually, 82 per cent severe to moderately; **77 per cent** reported headaches pre-menstrually, 74 per cent general increased appetite, 53 per cent heart pounding and 50 per cent dizziness and fainting.

### ** Geraldine's Story **

Geraldine is a 33-year-old mother of three who works as a nursing auxiliary. She had had PMT since 1983, after the birth of her third baby.

She had severe symptoms in all four categories. She felt 'possessed' pre-menstrually and hardly recognized herself. She was withdrawn from life and disgusted with her own behaviour. Her eating habits were particularly erratic pre-menstrually. In particular she craved chocolate, which she felt immensely guilty about.

57

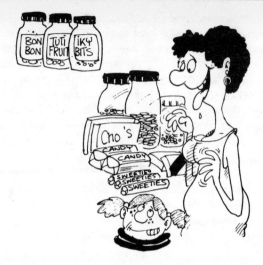

'I thought sometimes I could just sit zombie-like and not talk to anybody. I wanted to go to the doctor and ask him to take my children and put me in a white jacket and stick me in a room somewhere. In fact, it even makes me feel bad talking about it.

### Post-natal depression

When my third child was three months old I suddenly developed post-natal depression. It hit me really hard as I had never experienced it before. I didn't feel aggressive towards the baby, I just knew there was something wrong with me. I used to sit staring into space for hours. There were jobs that needed doing and the whole house was disintegrating, but I just couldn't do anything. I felt awful all the time and I had no energy or enthusiasm. I was overweight and depressed.

My doctor prescribed anti-depressants. I don't know if they helped or not. They helped me to sleep, but I was afraid I wouldn't wake up. They made me feel zombie-like.

I realized I had PMT during a sticky patch in my marriage. I felt I was reacting to everything and that some problem had to be present in order to make me feel so bad.

### Black cloud overhead

Whereas I hadn't felt aggressive with post-natal depression, I felt absolutely horrendous when I had PMT. I used to feel I had an individual black cloud *hanging over me. I'd wake up in the morning knowing that awful feeling was there and that there was nothing I could do to make it go away. I just knew I had days ahead of me feeling so awful.*

*I didn't want to participate in my usual activities pre-menstrually. I belong to an amateur dramatics society, but I just didn't feel I could do anything like that. You need to give a lot of yourself in things like that, and I didn't feel capable of doing what I was supposed to do. My memory just went, and I would literally go blank, and that applied to everything, not just my drama.*

*I felt like a zombie and wanted to withdraw from life. I was disgusted with my behaviour towards the children, who, as a result, are quite afraid of me. To compensate I'd then eat vast quantities of chocolate for comfort which would only serve to make my symptoms worse.*

*I often found myself hiding away to eat in private. I found the amount I was eating an embarrassment. If you fancy a bar of chocolate you go off and buy one and that's fine. But I could eat four or five bars at once, and then eat the same amount again. You can't get rid of that many sweet papers. So you gradually ease them out of your pocket, or wrap them in something else, and throw them in the bin. The children would notice I'd had more than one bar; I couldn't pull the wool over their eyes. I wasn't aware that I was being silly at the time, I just used to sit and eat and then feel so sick afterwards.*

*I knew I wouldn't do any housework in the days to come, and that I wouldn't want to do anything with the children. I would be unbearable to my husband and I wouldn't bother to cook.*

*My doctor again prescribed anti-depressants. But knowing they made me feel zombie-like, I didn't want to take them any more. I was also prescribed diuretics. Unfortunately they seem to stop my bladder working properly, because I can't make it to the loo in time. So they were really out anyway.*

*I also tried vitamin B6, evening primrose oil, multi-vitamins, ginseng and progesterone pessaries.*

*At the time I felt life wasn't really worth living. I existed from situation to situation. It was a very stressful time. I had one good week in four. It was unbearable for the family; it was really horrible. I thought I was going round the bend, totally insane and that no one could help me at all. I didn't really know who to contact as I'd tried all my doctor had to offer. I then read an article in a women's magazine about the nutritional approach to PMT and the work the Stewarts were doing.*

# PRE-MENSTRUAL SYNDROME QUESTIONNAIRE

Name: _Geraldine Ellis_          Age: _32_     Height: _5' 9"_     Weight: _10st 7lb_

MARITAL STATUS:      Single_____     Married__✓__     Divorced_____     Widowed_____
(Please tick where applicable)

PRESENT CONTRACEPTION:     None_____     Pill_____     I.U.D. _____     Other__✓__

   Your periods come every_ 28 _days     Your periods last_ 7–8 _days

   Your periods are:  Light_____     Moderate__✓__     Heavy_____

   Number of Pregnancies:_ 3 _     Number of Miscarriages:_____

Birth weight of children:  1st Child_7lb 3oz_   2nd Child_8lb 1oz_   3rd Child_8lb 11oz_   4th Child_____

| SYMPTOMS | WEEK AFTER PERIOD (Fill in 3 days after period) | | | | WEEK BEFORE PERIOD (Fill in 2-3 days before period) | | | |
|---|---|---|---|---|---|---|---|---|
| | None | Mild | Moderate | Severe | None | Mild | Moderate | Severe |
| **PMT - A** | | | | | | | | |
| Nervous Tension | ✓ | | | | | ✓ | | |
| Mood Swings | ✓ | | | | | | ✓ | |
| Irritability | ✓ | | | | | | | ✓ |
| Anxiety | ✓ | | | | | ✓ | | |
| **PMT - H** | | | | | | | | |
| Weight gain | ✓ | | | | | ✓ | | |
| Swelling of Extremities | ✓ | | | | | | | ✓ |
| Breast Tenderness | ✓ | | | | | | ✓ | |
| Abdominal Bloating | ✓ | | | | | | ✓ | |
| **PMT - C** | | | | | | | | |
| Headache | ✓ | | | | | ✓ | | |
| Craving for Sweets | ✓ | | | | | | | ✓ |
| Increased Appetite | ✓ | | | | | | | ✓ |
| Heart Pounding | ✓ | | | | | ✓ | | |
| Fatigue | ✓ | | | | | | | ✓ |
| Dizziness or Fainting | ✓ | | | | | ✓ | | |
| **PMT - D** | | | | | | | | |
| Depression | ✓ | | | | | | | ✓ |
| Forgetfulness | ✓ | | | | | | ✓ | |
| Crying | ✓ | | | | | | | ✓ |
| Confusion | ✓ | | | | | | ✓ | |
| Insomnia | ✓ | | | | | ✓ | | |
| **OTHER SYMPTOMS** | | | | | | | | |
| Loss of Sexual Interest | ✓ | | | | | | | ✓ |
| Disorientation | ✓ | | | | | ✓ | | |
| Clumsiness | ✓ | | | | | | ✓ | |
| Tremors/Shakes | ✓ | | | | | ✓ | | |
| Thoughts of Suicide | ✓ | | | | | ✓ | | |
| Agoraphobia | ✓ | | | | | | | ✓ |
| Increased Physical Activity | ✓ | | | | | ✓ | | |
| Heavy/Aching Legs | ✓ | | | | | | ✓ | |
| Generalized Aches | ✓ | | | | | | ✓ | |
| Bad Breath | ✓ | | | | | ✓ | | |
| Sensitivity to Music/Light | ✓ | | | | | ✓ | | |
| Excessive Thirst | ✓ | | | | | ✓ | | |

One of Geraldine's particular weaknesses was her craving for sweet food premenstrually and her excessive indulgence. Later on in Chapter 11, I will be talking about the detrimental effects of excessive amounts of sweet food, particularly in relation to PMT symptoms.

On her first chart Geraldine's worst symptoms were in the sub-groups PMT C and PMT D, although she did have severe symptoms in all four categories.

Like the majority of women, Geraldine was lacking in education about the importance of a correct diet. This is hardly surprising considering how little we learned at school about nutrition as a subject. Until recent times very little attention has been placed on the role of nutrition in relation to women's health.

> *'I knew a bit about diet, but had no idea that changing my diet could bring me back to normal, and that's what it has done. Although I didn't know that I was sensitive to any foods, I had a good idea what was and what wasn't a sensible diet. My trouble was temptation. It's much easier to buy chocolate, which is available wherever you go, than it is to go home and make fish cakes with sesame seeds on them or things like that which you know are much better for you. I did eat healthy things, but I also ate a load of rubbish.*
>
> *I try to stick to the diet. I feel much better when I do. I know I shouldn't eat chocolates, processed food, salty food or wheat. I did try some Stilton cheese and crisps, but I blew up like a balloon shortly after eating them. I now know that chocolate makes me depressed, and of course I put on weight if I eat rubbish.*

### End result

> *Since I've been following the nutritional programme I feel so much better. My children notice the difference in me; I am no longer nasty to them. It has made me feel so much better in myself. I personally feel fine, although I could still do with losing weight.*
>
> *I still have my marital problems. But I know that we have got things wrong marriage-wise, I know they are not related to PMT. I haven't got that aggressiveness inside me so much and I haven't got that awful feeling, that black cloud hanging over my head. That was the worst thing.'*

Geraldine's follow-up chart verifies her story. Apart from a few remaining mild symptoms at the time of writing, she felt that she had overcome her PMT.

Another victim of chocolate cravings was Anita Walker. Her addiction to chocolate was no secret. It ran her life. She admits that she had little control over it. When you read her story, she could so easily be talking about a drug or alcohol.

# FOLLOW UP
## PRE-MENSTRUAL SYNDROME QUESTIONNAIRE

Name: _Geraldine Ellis_          Age: _32_     Height: _5' 9"_     Weight: _10st_

MARITAL STATUS:       Single_____     Married _✓_     Divorced_____     Widowed_____
(Please tick where applicable)

PRESENT CONTRACEPTION:       None_____     Pill_____     I.U.D._____     Other_✓_

　　　Your periods come every _28_ days       Your periods last _7–8_ days

　　　Your periods are:   Light_____       Moderate_✓_       Heavy_____

| SYMPTOMS | WEEK AFTER PERIOD (Fill in 3 days after period) | | | | WEEK BEFORE PERIOD (Fill in 2-3 days before period) | | | |
|---|---|---|---|---|---|---|---|---|
| | None | Mild | Moderate | Severe | None | Mild | Moderate | Severe |
| **PMT - A** | | | | | | | | |
| Nervous Tension | ✓ | | | | ✓ | | | |
| Mood Swings | ✓ | | | | ✓ | | | |
| Irritability | ✓ | | | | ✓ | | | |
| Anxiety | ✓ | | | | ✓ | | | |
| **PMT - H** | | | | | | | | |
| Weight gain | ✓ | | | | | ✓ | | |
| Swelling of Extremities | ✓ | | | | ✓ | | | |
| Breast Tenderness | ✓ | | | | ✓ | | | |
| Abdominal Bloating | ✓ | | | | | ✓ | | |
| **PMT - C** | | | | | | | | |
| Headache | ✓ | | | | ✓ | | | |
| Craving for Sweets | ✓ | | | | | ✓ | | |
| Increased Appetite | ✓ | | | | ✓ | | | |
| Heart Pounding | ✓ | | | | ✓ | | | |
| Fatigue | ✓ | | | | ✓ | | | |
| Dizziness or Fainting | ✓ | | | | ✓ | | | |
| **PMT - D** | | | | | | | | |
| Depression | ✓ | | | | ✓ | | | |
| Forgetfulness | ✓ | | | | ✓ | | | |
| Crying | ✓ | | | | ✓ | | | |
| Confusion | ✓ | | | | ✓ | | | |
| Insomnia | ✓ | | | | ✓ | | | |
| **OTHER SYMPTOMS** | | | | | | | | |
| Loss of Sexual Interest | ✓ | | | | ✓ | | | |
| Disorientation | ✓ | | | | ✓ | | | |
| Clumsiness | ✓ | | | | ✓ | | | |
| Tremors/Shakes | ✓ | | | | ✓ | | | |
| Thoughts of Suicide | ✓ | | | | ✓ | | | |
| Agoraphobia | ✓ | | | | ✓ | | | |
| Increased Physical Activity | ✓ | | | | ✓ | | | |
| Heavy/Aching Legs | ✓ | | | | ✓ | | | |
| Generalized Aches | ✓ | | | | ✓ | | | |
| Bad Breath | ✓ | | | | ✓ | | | |
| Sensitivity to Music/Light | ✓ | | | | ✓ | | | |
| Excessive Thirst | ✓ | | | | ✓ | | | |

## ANITA WALKER – SUGAR CRAVINGS

*'I am actually embarrassed to tell you about my sugar cravings. I would eat masses of chocolate bars, I could eat two bags of fun-size chocolate bars, or seven or eight ordinary bars and half a cake, and then eat my tea.*

*The more I ate, the worse my cravings would be, it was a vicious circle. I would feel OK for a bit after eating all that, and then I would feel awful. Especially more irritable, and especially more aggressive!*

*I didn't recognize that this was happening pre-menstrually at the time. I felt as though the toxins were building up and I would have to go to bed early, feeling fat and sick and having eaten myself into a stupor.'*

I'm hardly surprised that Anita felt embarrassed to relate this part of her story. She was a real 'chocoholic'. Fortunately, we were able to relieve her of these cravings early on in her programme. In the Self-Help section on page 169 I will explain how Anita also managed to overcome her thrush.

# 8

# DEPRESSION, CRYING AND THOUGHTS OF SUICIDE

## PMT D (DEPRESSION)

Fortunately, it is not common for women to suffer with PMT D alone. Such a patient would be in a highly depressed state, confused, even incoherent or feeling suicidal. She would probably not seek medical help herself, but would certainly be in urgent need of it. Where PMT D exists alone, it is vital that the patient receives good medical care.

It is more common for PMT D to be present together with PMT A. Usually the PMT A comes first and the feelings of depression, confusion, insomnia and outbursts of tears follow a few days before the onset of the period.

It is possible that the depressive symptoms of PMT D are related to a low oestrogen level. French workers have recently shown that women attempting suicide around the time of their period tended to have low oestrogen levels, but this was not universally the case. The cause for this is uncertain, but nutritional factors, stress and even lead in the environment are possibilities. Lead can apparently interfere with the way in which the body responds to oestrogen.

Certainly, lack of B vitamins has been described in depressed and anxious subjects, both in the United Kingdom and in the United States. However, simply giving some B vitamins is not usually the whole answer.

Depression is often linked with being overweight, and this we have observed in women contacting the WNAS. Those with bad PMT D tend to be more over-weight than those in other PMT sub-groups.

In our study we found that 94 per cent of the women suffered from pre-menstrual depression, 83.8 per cent severe to moderately. This, we felt, was a frighteningly high number, and in view of the possible consequences of depression, not something that should be taken lightly.

| Degree to which 1000 women suffered depression pre-menstrually | | | | |
| --- | --- | --- | --- | --- |
| *Not Affected* | *Mild* | *Moderate* | *Severe* | *Total Affected* |
| 6% | 10.2% | 29.9% | 53.9% - | 94% |

In 1959 Dr Katharina Dalton published a study in the *British Medical Journal* which showed that the time of admission to hospital of depressed patients coincided with the menstrual period, the pre-menstrual phase, and ovulation.

The balance of hormones – or whatever determines their balance, seems to be crucial in controlling mood. We are beginning to learn how diet and lifestyle can influence our hormones and our moods.

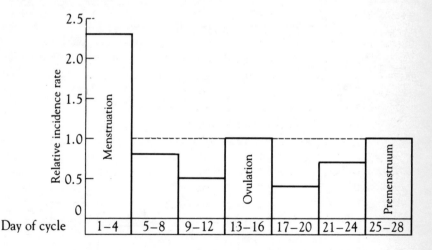

*Time of admission of 185 patients with depression. (From Dalton K. (1959). Br. Med. J.; 1:148–149.)*

65

## SUICIDAL

Many women who were suffering with PMT D reported that they felt suicidal, indeed it was because we were coming across so many women who felt suicidal that we decided to embark on the study of 1000 women.

Tragically, we found that 41 per cent of them had previously contemplated suicide pre-menstrually, 35 per cent of them several times and 5.8 per cent had actually attempted suicide pre-menstrually. That is a staggering 58 women out of 1000 that were chosen.

Conditions of the families of these women hardly bear thinking about. At this end of the scale it is a very sad and difficult problem indeed.

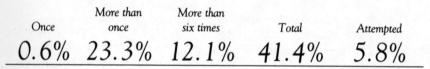

**Suicidal tendencies
out of a
sample of 1000 women**

| Once | *More than once* | *More than six times* | *Total* | *Attempted* |
|------|------|------|------|------|
| 0.6% | 23.3% | 12.1% | 41.4% | 5.8% |

Again in 1959 Dr Dalton looked at the timing of 276 acute psychiatric admissions in four London hospitals. According to her findings, which were published in the *British Medical Journal*, 46 per cent of the patients were admitted between the 25th day of their cycle and the 4th day of their new cycle.

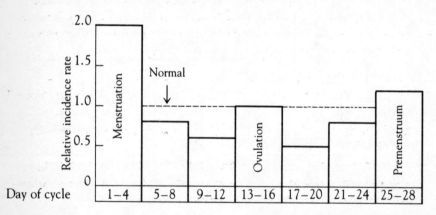

*Time of acute psychiatric admission in 276 patients. (From Dalton K. (1959). Br. Med. J.; 1:148–149.)*

Also 53 per cent of attempted suicides, 47 per cent of admissions for depression and 47 per cent of schizophrenic patients were admitted during these eight days of the menstrual cycle.

## " Sally's Story "

Sally is a 38-year-old woman who works as a recruitment consultant. She was married previously, but is now divorced.

Sally seriously contemplated taking a whole bottle of pills when she was pre-menstrual. Fortunately, she saw the light in time and relates the story to us as if she were talking about someone else.

'I really thought I was mentally ill, mentally inadequate; I thought I was cracking up. I was frightened to tell people how I felt because they might have thought I was a loony.

I did seriously contemplate suicide once. It was a bad time for me anyway as I was under a lot of stress. Being pre-menstrual was the last straw and I did contemplate taking a whole bottle of pills. Fortunately, I have some faith in God and I'm sure that's what eventually pulled me together and stopped me.

I felt that I was unbalanced and I couldn't stand the pain that the depression inside was causing any more. I just wanted to go to sleep so that it would all end.

PMT meant the pain of depression. I felt absolute despair pre-menstrually and I cannot express in words how desolate this made me feel. I really thought I was mentally ill. I thought my mind was taking over. Anything and everything was too stressful for me, and I felt I just couldn't cope.

### Stress
I would say stress definitely did influence my symptoms. When I was under stress I tended to get a runny tummy, therefore I don't suppose I got the full benefit of my food. It's like a vicious circle to me. When I'm under stress I don't eat, and then as a result I feel even more stressed.

However, since I have been following the programme I am definitely less affected by stress. I seem much more able to cope with stressful situations, which I certainly wouldn't have been able to cope with before.

I tried vitamin B6. It wasn't any help, but I think I know why. I discovered on the programme that I have a sensitivity to yeast, and the B6 tablets I was

67

*taking were yeast-based. I found that the B6 would perk me up and then I would drop down mentally and have a terrible bloated tummy.*

*I also tried evening primrose oil, which helped a little. I was prescribed anti-depressants, which were no help at all. They just made me feel out of control. They controlled a bit of the depression, but they just made me void of other emotions.*

*I didn't really recognize my symptoms as PMT. That was the worst thing, looking back. I just knew I was suffering with depression and agoraphobia regularly, in fact towards the end most of the time. I only had one good week after my period, the rest of the time was distressing. When I first saw the Women's Nutritional Advisory Service questionnaire and realized that agoraphobic symptoms could be part of the Pre-Menstrual Syndrome it gave me a great sense of relief. I felt a bit better just knowing that my symptoms were part of PMT. It gave me a far greater understanding of my suffering.*

*I thought I would give the nutritional approach to PMT a try as I felt so unwell, and I was so sick of taking anti-depressants and sleeping tablets. I had to do something as I honestly felt I was cracking up.'*

Imagine having to live with the secret that you thought you were mentally ill. As a divorcee, Sally had to fend for herself.

Her job and her income were exceedingly important and she obviously thought these were threatened by her severe symptoms. She had tried several solutions, like our other patients, but did not find her symptoms lessened.

She suffered pre-menstrually with severe symptoms in all four categories, as her chart shows. She also had pre-menstrual agoraphobia, which was a terrific handicap in her working and social life.

### The power of diet

*'I used to eat lots of bread, cakes, animal fats including lots of butter and drink a substantial amount of tea and coffee.*

*I had no idea that my symptoms could be diet-related until I read an article in a magazine. I realized at that point that it was likely that something in my diet might be making me feel so bad.*

*The diet recommended was a bit bewildering at first, probably because it's so different. I was asked to come off grains for a short period, and to omit all foods with a yeast base from my diet. I had to cut down my junk food intake, including sugary foods, i.e. biscuits, cakes, puddings. Also to cut down on salt, alcohol and dairy products.*

68

## PRE-MENSTRUAL SYNDROME QUESTIONNAIRE

Name: _Sally Noone_____ Age: _38___ Height: _5′ 3″___ Weight: _9st_____

MARITAL STATUS: Single_____ Married_____ Divorced___✓__ Widowed_____
(Please tick where applicable)

PRESENT CONTRACEPTION: None_____ Pill_____ I.U.D. _____ Other___✓___

    Your periods come every _29_____ days    Your periods last____3____ days

    Your periods are: Light_____ Moderate___✓_____ Heavy_____

    Number of Pregnancies:____–_____ Number of Miscarriages:_____–_____

Birth weight of children: 1st Child_____ 2nd Child_____ 3rd Child_____ 4th Child_____

| SYMPTOMS | WEEK AFTER PERIOD (Fill in 3 days after period) | | | | WEEK BEFORE PERIOD (Fill in 2-3 days before period) | | | |
|---|---|---|---|---|---|---|---|---|
| | None | Mild | Moderate | Severe | None | Mild | Moderate | Severe |
| **PMT - A** | | | | | | | | |
| Nervous Tension | | | ✓ | | | | | ✓ |
| Mood Swings | | | ✓ | | | | | ✓ |
| Irritability | | | ✓ | | | | | ✓ |
| Anxiety | | | ✓ | | | | | ✓ |
| **PMT - H** | | | | | | | | |
| Weight gain | ✓ | | | | | | | ✓ |
| Swelling of Extremities | ✓ | | | | | ✓ | | |
| Breast Tenderness | ✓ | | | | | | ✓ | |
| Abdominal Bloating | | ✓ | | | | | | ✓ |
| **PMT - C** | | | | | | | | |
| Headache | | ✓ | | | | ✓ | | |
| Craving for Sweets | ✓ | | | | | | | ✓ |
| Increased Appetite | ✓ | | | | | | | ✓ |
| Heart Pounding | | ✓ | | | | | | ✓ |
| Fatigue | | | ✓ | | | | | ✓ |
| Dizziness or Fainting | ✓ | | | | | | | ✓ |
| **PMT - D** | | | | | | | | |
| Depression | | ✓ | | | | | | ✓ |
| Forgetfulness | | ✓ | | | | | | ✓ |
| Crying | | | ✓ | | | | | ✓ |
| Confusion | | ✓ | | | | | | ✓ |
| Insomnia | | ✓ | | | | | | ✓ |
| **OTHER SYMPTOMS** | | | | | | | | |
| Loss of Sexual Interest | | | | ✓ | | | | ✓ |
| Disorientation | | ✓ | | | | | | ✓ |
| Clumsiness | | ✓ | | | | | ✓ | |
| Tremors/Shakes | ✓ | | | | | | | ✓ |
| Thoughts of Suicide | ✓ | | | | | | | ✓ |
| Agoraphobia | ✓ | | | | | | | ✓ |
| Increased Physical Activity | ✓ | | | | | | | ✓ |
| Heavy/Aching Legs | | ✓ | | | | ✓ | | |
| Generalized Aches | | ✓ | | | | | ✓ | |
| Bad Breath | ✓ | | | | | | | ✓ |
| Sensitivity to Music/Light | ✓ | | | | | | | ✓ |
| Excessive Thirst | ✓ | | | | | | | ✓ |

*I soon got used to the diet. In fact I feel I have now revamped my whole way of eating, and I enjoy my food more. I found that I have a sensitivity to wheat, sugar and chocolate. If I eat them I get a reaction the next day. I get a mild sort of dizziness and windy stomach. I know now that it is going to be over within 24 hours, whereas before I would get so upset and confused because I wouldn't know what was causing it. To tell the truth, when my tummy used to swell, I really thought I had cancer.*

*My symptoms disappeared on the programme. The depression cleared within one week and the remaining symptoms gradually disappeared during the first three months. So much so, I decided I no longer needed to follow the recommendations. Coming off the diet and reverting to my previous diet brought the symptoms back. I went back on to the programme recommended, and within a short space of time my symptoms were under control again. I've proved to myself that the diet works for me.*

*I have been taking Optivite since I started the programme. That and the diet have done so much good for me. I really think that Optivite is the best thing since sliced bread.*

### End result

*Now that I have been through the programme, I am much more stable. I am able to stick at my job and maintain my concentration. I have a very stressful job, but I am now able to work hard and I feel very happy. PMT does not affect me now. The programme has changed my life. I can cope better with everything. I would say I am a thousand times better. I no longer feel exhausted after little effort. I am so delighted. Looking back, it's like looking at a different person.'*

Once again you can see that Sally's symptoms have gone from severe to mild in just a few months. She feels her life has returned to normal because she followed the nutritional programme, which is reflected in her final chart and letter as follows.

*Dear Maryon,*

*I am writing to let you know that there is a marked change in my life. I feel that I have come through the proverbial 'long dark tunnel' out of despair into sunlight. If only I had known about the yeast allergy years ago and trusted my instinct about magnesium, the before and after picture shown on the symptom tables would not have been so acutely marked!*

*I think because I had hidden all the symptoms and bottled them up, my family are not really aware of the change I feel inside. There was certainly scepticism from one branch of my family when I tried to explain it to them, and*

# FOLLOW UP
## PRE-MENSTRUAL SYNDROME QUESTIONNAIRE

Name: __Sally Noone__          Age: __38__      Height: __5' 3"__      Weight: __8st 9lb__

MARITAL STATUS:     Single __✓__     Married _____     Divorced _____     Widowed _____
(Please tick where applicable)

PRESENT CONTRACEPTION:     None __✓__  Pill _____  I.U.D. _____     Other _____

   Your periods come every __28__ days     Your periods last __3__ days

   Your periods are:   Light _____     Moderate __✓__     Heavy _____

| SYMPTOMS | WEEK AFTER PERIOD (Fill in 3 days after period) | | | | WEEK BEFORE PERIOD (Fill in 2-3 days before period) | | | |
|---|---|---|---|---|---|---|---|---|
| | None | Mild | Moderate | Severe | None | Mild | Moderate | Severe |
| **PMT - A** | | | | | | | | |
| Nervous Tension | ✓ | | | | | ✓ | | |
| Mood Swings | ✓ | | | | ✓ | | | |
| Irritability | ✓ | | | | | | ✓ | |
| Anxiety | ✓ | | | | | ✓ | | |
| **PMT - H** | | | | | | | | |
| Weight gain | ✓ | | | | ✓ | | | |
| Swelling of Extremities | ✓ | | | | ✓ | | | |
| Breast Tenderness | ✓ | | | | | | ✓ | |
| Abdominal Bloating | ✓ | | | | | | ✓ | |
| **PMT - C** | | | | | | | | |
| Headache | ✓ | | | | ✓ | | | |
| Craving for Sweets | ✓ | | | | | | ✓ | |
| Increased Appetite | ✓ | | | | ✓ | | | |
| Heart Pounding | ✓ | | | | ✓ | | | |
| Fatigue | ✓ | | | | | ✓ | | |
| Dizziness or Fainting | ✓ | | | | ✓ | | | |
| **PMT - D** | | | | | | | | |
| Depression | ✓ | | | | | ✓ | | |
| Forgetfulness | ✓ | | | | ✓ | | | |
| Crying | ✓ | | | | ✓ | | | |
| Confusion | ✓ | | | | ✓ | | | |
| Insomnia | ✓ | | | | ✓ | | | |
| **OTHER SYMPTOMS** | | | | | | | | |
| Loss of Sexual Interest | | ✓ | | | ✓ | | | |
| Disorientation | ✓ | | | | ✓ | | | |
| Clumsiness | ✓ | | | | | | ✓ | |
| Tremors/Shakes | ✓ | | | | ✓ | | | |
| Thoughts of Suicide | ✓ | | | | ✓ | | | |
| Agoraphobia | ✓ | | | | ✓ | | | |
| Increased Physical Activity | ✓ | | | | ✓ | | | |
| Heavy/Aching Legs | ✓ | | | | ✓ | | | |
| Generalized Aches | ✓ | | | | ✓ | | | |
| Bad Breath | ✓ | | | | ✓ | | | |
| Sensitivity to Music/Light | ✓ | | | | ✓ | | | |
| Excessive Thirst | ✓ | | | | ✓ | | | |

*why I was being 'faddish' about my food. The knowledge that certain foods will send me back into the downward spiral of depression is enough to ensure that I steer clear of any of them, and keep to the new regime.*

*I am getting to be a bore with some of my friends. As soon as they start complaining about any of the symptoms I used to have, I try to analyse their diet for them and I also give them your address – whether they want it or not!*

*I do hope you manage to get the message across to all the women who need it – for anyone else to suffer the way I did, and not to know the way out – well, it is criminal and so much more must be done.*

    *Sally Noone*
    *(a convert)*

PMT D can be very severe indeed. We have dealt with some very sad cases, where women felt suicidal, depressed and that life was not worth living pre-menstrually. The first example I will give you is the story of Anita Walker.

## " Anita's Story "

Anita is a 36-year-old mother of two children who works as personnel assistant. Her PMT began when she was seventeen years old, but became worse about eight years ago after having children and a miscarriage. She has also had a hysterectomy due to excessive bleeding and fibroids.

*'I ended up with only four or five normal days per month. The rest of the time, apart from my period, I'd get fatter and fatter. I'd feel tired and irritable and couldn't concentrate, to the point where I didn't know what day of the week it was.*

*I attacked my husband with a knife on several occasions. I kept away from the baby as I was terrified of baby battering; I knew I could so easily have done it.*

*I remember feeling suicidal and not knowing where I was. I'd find myself out in the street yelling in the middle of the night, this happened pre-menstrually. It was like being Jekyll and Hyde. I'd be totally irrational and make stupid decisions. The week after, I'd look back and wonder why on earth I acted that way.*

*One night, a week before my period, feeling nobody cared, I thought I just couldn't go on any more. I felt fat, depressed and I didn't think life was worth living for a week to ten days before my period. I was utterly desperate. I got this bottle of wine and my nice collection of sleeping pills that my doctor had doled out.*

*I just quietly swallowed the lot, and the next thing I knew I was waking up in hospital, wondering what I was doing there.*

*No connection was made there between my condition and PMT. They just told me to go away, not to be a silly girl, and to stop upsetting my family. No treatment offered by my doctor made any lasting impact on my symptoms.*

### What about me?

*I never liked myself pre-menstrually. I really did feel worthless as a human being. I was aware that eating junk food and giving in to my cravings made me far worse. If I had some "sinful" foods in the cupboard I would eat them all pre-menstrually, and then tell myself that I deserved to feel awful, because that was all I was fit for. It felt like I was punishing myself. I felt utterly fatigued. I'd go to bed at 8 p.m. each night, feeling dead, and then wake up the next morning feeling equally awful.*

*I always used to feel I wasn't doing my job properly. I think I inherited this from my mother. Looking back I think she suffered too. There were times when my father would come home to find us throwing things around the kitchen at each other. We'd be fine for a couple of weeks and then it would all start up again.*

### What about them?

*I really hated everybody when I was pre-menstrual. I used to turn my anger onto myself as I couldn't bear to see the effect it had on others. I felt like I literally changed character, like Jekyll and Hyde.*

*The suicidal feelings I had were both strange and positive. I couldn't talk myself out of them, despite the fact that I really knew, deep down, that suicide was not a good solution. I felt so determined at times, I really felt I would have succeeded if I hadn't been found.*

*I must emphasize that these feelings and suicidal tendencies only occurred pre-menstrually. I felt utterly dreadful pre-menstrually, like a jibbering wreck.*

*I think stress aggravated the situation. Both my husband and I are in high-pressure jobs. I've been attending relaxation classes which I find helpful. I don't find it easy to unwind; there is a part of me that remains burning away, probably because I tend to lack confidence and so I'm always pushing myself. I used to burn out at PMT times, but I don't any more.*

*Apart from all the drugs and sleeping tablets I was given, I also tried diuretics, which were prescribed by my doctor as I used to put on seven pounds*

*(3 kg) pre-menstrually. They helped a little bit initially, but by the end of the day my symptoms would be back and I felt as if I was getting nowhere.*

*My doctor then prescribed Primolut N in massive doses and all it succeeded in doing was make me gain even more weight. There was a time, five or six years ago, when I tried hormone treatment, but I didn't get on very well with that either. I felt I was given too much, and it seemed to exaggerate my symptoms. I had a Well Woman test at the time and they said how enlarged my uterus was, and that it was probably due to the hormones.*

*It was through the media that I learned about the nutritional approach to PMT.'*

Anita was a classic case of pure PMT. She had practically no symptoms after her period, and very severe symptoms in all four sub-categories of PMT pre-menstrually, which you can see on her first chart.

Again, from the sound of her symptoms she might well have been classified as a psychiatric patient. After all, screaming in the street in the middle of the night and suicidal feelings are not classified as socially acceptable behaviour.

Although she was taking prescribed sleeping tablets and hormones, she was unable to function properly. Consequently she found it unbelievably difficult to keep herself together at work. It was a wonder she managed to hold down her job at all under the circumstances. You can see how severe these symptoms were from her first chart.

*'When I began the nutritional PMT programme, I was taking both Primolut N and Mogadon. Very soon after I was able to stop taking both of the drugs. I no longer felt I needed them.*

### The new diet

*I made all the dietary changes suggested and stuck to them rigidly. In fact, I changed the whole family's diet. My son turned out to have some allergies which had been causing behavioural problems. My husband also turned out to have a problem. One day when he was under a lot of stress, he went out to lunch. He ate a lot of bread and pasta and had some alcohol with the meal. On the train on the way home his bladder stopped working and an ambulance had to be called as he was in a terrible state of near-collapse. He was rushed to hospital and was subsequently diagnosed as having a massive dose of thrush. He said it was the most awful thing in his life, the swelling and the irritation were so bad.*

*I took him off wheat and yeast-based foods and I am now very particular about our diet.*

74

## PRE-MENSTRUAL SYNDROME QUESTIONNAIRE

Name: __Anita Walker__    Age: __36__    Height: __5′ 4½″__    Weight: __11st__

MARITAL STATUS:    Single _____    Married __✓__    Divorced _____    Widowed _____
(Please tick where applicable)

PRESENT CONTRACEPTION:    None _____    Pill _____    I.U.D. __✓__    Other _____

Your periods come every __28__ days    Your periods last __7__ days

Your periods are:    Light _____    Moderate _____    Heavy __✓__

Number of Pregnancies: __4__    Number of Miscarriages: __2__

Birth weight of children:    1st Child __7lb 3oz__    2nd Child __8lb 2oz__    3rd Child _____    4th Child _____

| SYMPTOMS | WEEK AFTER PERIOD (Fill in 3 days after period) | | | | WEEK BEFORE PERIOD (Fill in 2-3 days before period) | | | |
|---|---|---|---|---|---|---|---|---|
|  | None | Mild | Moderate | Severe | None | Mild | Moderate | Severe |
| **PMT - A** | | | | | | | | |
| Nervous Tension | ✓ | | | | | | | ✓ |
| Mood Swings | ✓ | | | | | | | ✓ |
| Irritability | ✓ | | | | | | | ✓ |
| Anxiety | ✓ | | | | | | | ✓ |
| **PMT - H** | | | | | | | | |
| Weight gain | ✓ | | | | | | | ✓ |
| Swelling of Extremities | | | ✓ | | | | | ✓ |
| Breast Tenderness | ✓ | | | | | | | ✓ |
| Abdominal Bloating | | ✓ | | | | | | ✓ |
| **PMT - C** | | | | | | | | |
| Headache | ✓ | | | | | ✓ | | |
| Craving for Sweets | ✓ | | | | | | | ✓ |
| Increased Appetite | ✓ | | | | | | | ✓ |
| Heart Pounding | ✓ | | | | ✓ | | | |
| Fatigue | ✓ | | | | | | | ✓ |
| Dizziness or Fainting | ✓ | | | | ✓ | | | |
| **PMT - D** | | | | | | | | |
| Depression | ✓ | | | | | | | ✓ |
| Forgetfulness | ✓ | | | | | | | ✓ |
| Crying | ✓ | | | | | | ✓ | |
| Confusion | ✓ | | | | | | | ✓ |
| Insomnia | ✓ | | | | | | | ✓ |
| **OTHER SYMPTOMS** | | | | | | | | |
| Loss of Sexual Interest | ✓ | | | | | ✓ | | |
| Disorientation | ✓ | | | | | | | ✓ |
| Clumsiness | ✓ | | | | | | | ✓ |
| Tremors/Shakes | ✓ | | | | | | | ✓ |
| Thoughts of Suicide | ✓ | | | | | | | ✓ |
| Agoraphobia | ✓ | | | | | ✓ | | |
| Increased Physical Activity | ✓ | | | | ✓ | | | |
| Heavy/Aching Legs | ✓ | | | | | | | ✓ |
| Generalized Aches | ✓ | | | | | | | ✓ |
| Bad Breath | ✓ | | | | | | | ✓ |
| Sensitivity to Music/Light | ✓ | | | | ✓ | | | |
| Excessive Thirst | ✓ | | | | | | | ✓ |

*The whole family now look and feel better. You can see it, they sort of "glow" somehow. They are not black around the eyes as they used to be, their hair shines and they have a lot more energy. Maybe that's partly because they have a lot more green vegetables and other fresh raw foods.*

*We now watch each other's plates and occasionally, if he's suspicious, Mark, my son, will check through my bag!*

### Come home Mum, all is forgiven

*We can actually hold a conversation now. We have good discussions and I really think my family are coming around to thinking I'm a worthwhile person again, probably because I myself consider I am. I can actually say we do have a normal married life now. David is delighted we live life normally and feels it's great that we are still together, which is lovely. We all joke about my former behaviour. They are much more responsive now, but then again I suppose I am, too.'*

After six months Anita had her PMT well and truly under control. She had some remaining mild symptoms which she finds comparatively easy to live with – although within another few months these too should disappear.

The comparison between her two questionnaires clearly shows the progress that Anita felt she made during the six months on the programme, and her letter outlines how her life has since changed.

*Dear Maryon,*

*A very big thank-you to your team for saving a life and a marriage.*

*As you know, when I wrote to you, I had tried everything I knew and everything my doctor knew to relieve the pain of my PMT. So I wrote to you and will always be glad I did, as the nutritional programme helped so much.*

*I felt that the hysterectomy without the nutritional programme would not have made such a difference. I can be certain that my speedy recovery was certainly thanks to good nutrition and definitely to the vitamin supplement, Optivite; I took six a day then.*

*When I wrote to you my only fear was 'What if this fails too?' I almost didn't post the letter when I contemplated the consequences of this: certain divorce, Ben taking the children away because of my emotional instability (and I would have agreed with him) and my certain self-destruction. Happily we can be sure now that this will not happen. As I said, you saved a life and marriage.*

*Whoever said 'you are what you eat' was so right. I do tend to think I am*

# FOLLOW UP
## PRE-MENSTRUAL SYNDROME QUESTIONNAIRE

Name: _Anita Walker_     Age: _36_     Height: _5' 4½"_     Weight: _10st 12lb_

MARITAL STATUS:     Single_____     Married__✓__     Divorced_____     Widowed_____
(Please tick where applicable)

PRESENT CONTRACEPTION:     None_____     Pill_____     I.U.D. __✓__     Other_____

Your periods come every _21_ days     Your periods last _7_ days

Your periods are:   Light_____     Moderate __✓__     Heavy_____

| SYMPTOMS | WEEK AFTER PERIOD (Fill in 3 days after period) | | | | WEEK BEFORE PERIOD (Fill in 2-3 days before period) | | | |
|---|---|---|---|---|---|---|---|---|
| | None | Mild | Moderate | Severe | None | Mild | Moderate | Severe |
| **PMT - A** | | | | | | | | |
| Nervous Tension | ✓ | | | | ✓ | | | |
| Mood Swings | ✓ | | | | | ✓ | | |
| Irritability | ✓ | | | | | ✓ | | |
| Anxiety | ✓ | | | | | ✓ | | |
| **PMT - H** | | | | | | | | |
| Weight gain | ✓ | | | | ✓ | | | |
| Swelling of Extremities | ✓ | | | | ✓ | | | |
| Breast Tenderness | ✓ | | | | ✓ | | | |
| Abdominal Bloating | ✓ | | | | ✓ | | | |
| **PMT - C** | | | | | | | | |
| Headache | ✓ | | | | | ✓ | | |
| Craving for Sweets | ✓ | | | | | ✓ | | |
| Increased Appetite | ✓ | | | | | ✓ | | |
| Heart Pounding | ✓ | | | | ✓ | | | |
| Fatigue | ✓ | | | | | ✓ | | |
| Dizziness or Fainting | ✓ | | | | ✓ | | | |
| **PMT - D** | | | | | | | | |
| Depression | ✓ | | | | ✓ | | | |
| Forgetfulness | ✓ | | | | ✓ | | | |
| Crying | ✓ | | | | ✓ | | | |
| Confusion | ✓ | | | | ✓ | | | |
| Insomnia | ✓ | | | | | | ✓ | |
| **OTHER SYMPTOMS** | | | | | | | | |
| Loss of Sexual Interest | ✓ | | | | ✓ | | | |
| Disorientation | ✓ | | | | | ✓ | | |
| Clumsiness | ✓ | | | | | ✓ | | |
| Tremors/Shakes | ✓ | | | | ✓ | | | |
| Thoughts of Suicide | ✓ | | | | ✓ | | | |
| Agoraphobia | ✓ | | | | ✓ | | | |
| Increased Physical Activity | ✓ | | | | ✓ | | | |
| Heavy/Aching Legs | ✓ | | | | ✓ | | | |
| Generalized Aches | ✓ | | | | ✓ | | | |
| Bad Breath | ✓ | | | | ✓ | | | |
| Sensitivity to Music/Light | ✓ | | | | ✓ | | | |
| Excessive Thirst | ✓ | | | | ✓ | | | |

*cured and slip back occasionally to bad eating habits. I then feel tired, cross and lethargic. I suffer this for a day or two and say, look, you're 'going-off' again, you're not cured at all. Then I realize what's happening, check back on what I've eaten, and within 36 hours can be all right again; the power of food!*

*I do enjoy the 'high' of constant energy and health and most of all the joy of not having to take drugs. I will recommend your Service to all who have difficulties. I am battling with my GP at present to recommend his patients to you but he sees it all as 'black magic'. He says I'm better because I think I'm better! He's only got to read my notes. The only time I have seen him since my hysterectomy last year was to talk to him about you. I have not consulted him for anything else.*

*Again, my thanks and that of my family*

*Anita Walker*

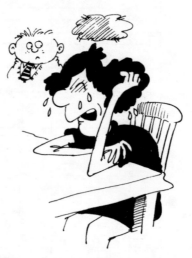

## PAULINE'S SUICIDAL FEELINGS

*'One day I felt so awful. I had pre-menstrual insomnia and was desperate to get some sleep. I decided I was going to have a good long sleep. I took all the tablets and then after a while I became panic-stricken and chickened out. I called my husband and told him what I'd done. I can't remember much, except he was trying to keep me awake. When the doctor arrived he said "We've had problems with you threatening to do this before, haven't we? It's your periods isn't it, you always get like that." This was because I'd said I felt like doing it many times in the past.'*

# 9

# OTHER SYMPTOMS – CLUMSINESS, LOSS OF SEX DRIVE AND AGORAPHOBIA

After the first year of providing nutritional help to women, it became obvious that there were other pre-menstrual symptoms that were affecting them severely. We made additions to the chart to assess the most common extra symptoms.

| | WEEK BEFORE PERIOD | | | | WEEK AFTER PERIOD | | | |
|---|---|---|---|---|---|---|---|---|
| OTHER SYMPTOMS | | | | | | | | |
| Loss of Sexual Interest | ✓ | | | | ✓ | | | |
| Disorientation | ✓ | | | | ✓ | | | |
| Clumsiness | ✓ | | | | ✓ | | | |
| Tremors/Shakes | ✓ | | | | ✓ | | | |
| Thoughts of Suicide | ✓ | | | | ✓ | | | |
| Agoraphobia | ✓ | | | | ✓ | | | |
| Increased Physical Activity | ✓ | | | | ✓ | | | |
| Heavy/Aching Legs | ✓ | | | | ✓ | | | |
| Generalized Aches | ✓ | | | | ✓ | | | |
| Bad Breath | ✓ | | | | ✓ | | | |
| Sensitivity to Music/Light | ✓ | | | | ✓ | | | |
| Excessive Thirst | ✓ | | | | ✓ | | | |

Do you have any other PRE-MENSTRUAL SYMPTOMS not listed above?

1. _____

2. _____

3. _____

4. _____

5. How much weight do you gain before your period? _____

## CLUMSINESS

Clumsiness was the most troublesome additional symptom to our 1000 patients outside the four sub-groups. Eighty-three per cent of sufferers reported being clumsy pre-menstrually, nearly 56 per cent severe to moderately.

The cause of pre-menstrual clumsiness is uncertain, but it may reflect a disturbance in the finer aspects of nervous system function, which might occur pre-menstrually. This can be caused by changes in brain chemistry, hormonal chemistry, lack of certain nutrients, excessive intake of tea, coffee, cigarettes or alcohol. The presence of pre-menstrual clumsiness suggests that there may well be a substantial physical, rather than psychological, component to such women's pre-menstrual symptoms.

**Degree to which clumsiness affected a sample of 1000 women pre-menstrually**

| None | Mild | Moderate | Severe | Total Affected |
|------|------|----------|--------|----------------|
| 16.6% | 27.5% | 36.1% | 19.8% | - 83.4% |

## SEX DRIVE

Out of a sample of 1000 PMT sufferers with sexual relationships 67 per cent reported decreased interest in sex and frequency of sexual intercourse pre-menstrually. Only 1.5 per cent reported increased sexual activity pre-menstrually.

We were concerned to see such a large number of women reporting similar distressing problems, so we decided to follow the progress of a group of 50 severe PMT sufferers, who also had severely decreased sex drive, through a three-month diet and supplement programme to see whether there was any improvement.

After three months these women were asked whether their interest in sex had altered. Fifty per cent of them reported that there had been a complete return to their libido (sex drive) and a further 38 per cent reported a significant but not full improvement to their libido. Only 12 per cent reported no change in libido at all.

The results were obviously very encouraging. Considering neither we nor the women had anticipated improvement in this area initially, it was considered by all to be an added bonus. In most cases the women did not associate their decreased libido with their PMT, and furthermore did not feel that reduced libido was a symptom, but merely a reflection of the state and stage of their relationship. Needless to say, many husbands and partners were satisfied with this particular result.

**Improvement in sex drive
of 50 women who had
previously reported a decrease**

| Little or no improvement | Significant but not full return to libido | Complete return of libido | | Total improvement |
|---|---|---|---|---|
| 12% | 38% | 50% | - | 88% |

## " Geraldine's Story "

Geraldine, who explained about her intense chocolate craving problems in the PMT C section, also feels her problems with her relationships and sex life were magnified because of her symptoms.

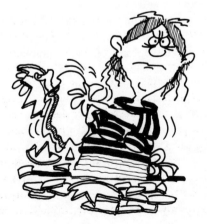

*'My relationship with my husband was definitely affected by my pre-menstrual symptoms. I think, in all fairness, we began going through a sticky patch before I had any of the symptoms, but in those days I didn't lash out and hit him. I'd just get worked up. With PMT I just started hitting out in anger. About the most frustrating thing is that he wouldn't row back. He'd just go quiet and go off, we could never discuss it.*

*I didn't want him to come anywhere near me pre-menstrually, let alone sexually. I didn't want him to cuddle me, touch me, talk to me or be there. I'd go right into myself and would really rather not have any contact with anyone at all.*

*A lot of the problems with my husband stem from PMT. I'd feel much worse than crabby, it was unbelievably horrible. The other issues would creep in once I'd started to get worked up, and it became very complex.'*

## AGORAPHOBIA

On our extended symptom list is the condition of agoraphobia, the exaggerated fear of going out alone. This was eventually added to the list as it seemed to be mentioned far more often than we had anticipated. At about this time we were contacted by a marvellous lady who was running a national group for agoraphobic sufferers. She had some amazing facts and figures about agoraphobia, including statistics on the incidence of PMT-suffering agoraphobic women.

Firstly, we were surprised to learn that 88 per cent of agoraphobia sufferers are women. Out of a sample of 94 agoraphobic women 91 per cent also suffered with PMT!

By coincidence, we had several severe PMT sufferers who also suffered severely with agoraphobia on our programme at this time. Many of them were making excellent progress, not only with the overcoming of their PMT symptoms, but their agoraphobia had also disappeared on the programme.

I'll never forget one joyous phone call I had from a lady in Jersey, who had taken herself out for the day for the first time in eight years. She had gone to have her hair permed and buy some clothes.

As she had previously only gone out accompanied by her husband or a neighbour, when her husband arrived home and found her missing he became understandably worried. After a while he began knocking on neighbours' doors to see whether she had gone visiting. By the time she casually wandered home her husband and neighbours were out in the street looking for her. They couldn't believe her new hair-do, and her husband wasn't sure whether to laugh or cry when he saw how many packages she had! He told me she's been costing him a fortune in evening entertainment ever since! Well, she has got eight years to make up for.

Agoraphobia is a very nasty condition: being afraid to go out is both anti-social and isolating for the victim, and can place an awful strain on a family. Here is the story of a woman who had been perfectly well until she underwent surgery for the purpose of sterilization. The change in her health was so unexpected that it had dramatic repercussions on her life.

## " Jane's Story "

Jane was a 36-year-old mother of three children who was trying to work part time at the time she contacted the Women's Nutritional Advisory Service. I say 'trying to work' as for six years she had been severely agoraphobic pre-menstrually.

*'It was six years ago that I went to my front door and discovered I couldn't walk through it. I was pre-menstrual at the time, and had noticed symptoms had begun after my sterilization.*

*I couldn't go out alone, not to the shops or to the bingo, which I had always taken in my stride. I really thought I was suffering from a very serious illness. I saw my doctor and he diagnosed nervous tension. I didn't believe him though, because I'm not the nervous type.*

*My doctor prescribed Valium, but it was no help. In fact it made me feel worse because it gave me panic attacks. I was on Valium for six months and then had great difficulty stopping. I went back to the doctor when I was pre-menstrual and just threw the tablets at him. I told him to never, ever prescribe me any kind of tablets like that again, as they made me feel so ill.*

*Previously, I would have been described by my family and friends as practical, hard-working and always full of fun and laughter. I was frightened and bewildered by the changes in myself. I found myself losing new friends as they grew tired of hearing my constant tales of woe.*

*I was at the doctor's every other week with my list of symptoms. He referred me to a psychiatrist at one point who insisted I was as strong as a horse and that the condition was all in my mind. I was gaining four to five pounds (2–3 kg) in weight pre-menstrually, suffering with severe breast soreness, pounding headaches, edginess and irritability and then the agoraphobia would start. I was sure it wasn't all in my mind.*

83

*After recovering from the effects of the Valium I had been taking, we decided to move so that I could be near my supportive family. My new doctor suggested hormone therapy as he said it was usually prescribed for women who were going through the menopause early, but I was only 36 years old! When I read contra-indications of the hormones I decided that as an overweight, over-35 smoker I should not be on these hormones.*

*I had now reached an impasse. My doctor had given his advice and I had refused to take it. Coincidentally, a few days later I saw an article in the newspaper about Maryon Stewart and the work she was doing at the Women's Nutritional Advisory Service. When I read the article I couldn't believe it. Here was someone describing me and my symptoms, saying that she had helped other people in similar situations.*

## I was like an old woman at 36

*I was suffering three out of every four weeks. I felt very uptight and niggly all the time. Plus I felt really frustrated and frightened that I couldn't get to the bottom of the problem.*

*The only way I could get out during the day was on the arm of an elderly neighbour in her seventies, who walks with the aid of a walking stick. There was I, half her age, clinging to her. Talk about the blind leading the blind! We'd even have to stop off on the way at my friend's shop because I was shaking so much.*

*I tried to forget it, but life was far from normal. I began to wonder if I would ever feel right again.*

## My miserable family

*I was sheer hell to live with. For five years I had lived a life of misery and so had my family. My husband was very good, considering what I put him through. I used to deliberately row with him pre-menstrually and pick holes in things. I was very agitated and always looking for an argument. He would avoid me at this time of my cycle. Sexual relations were a real problem in view of how I felt pre-menstrually, plus the fact that I was so tired, I just wasn't up to it.*

*My husband had to take me everywhere. I was utterly dependent on him. You can't have a normal relationship under these circumstances. But at least I am lucky that he was so supportive.'*

Jane's problem areas were PMT A, H and C as well as her agoraphobia. She was literally a shadow of her former self. Her 'before' and 'after' charts and a letter to us are here for you to examine. She also comments on the dietary changes she had to make on the nutritional programme.

*Dear Maryon,*

*As you know, when I first contacted you, I described all my symptoms of PMT. One was of being unable at certain times of the month (i.e. just before and after each period) to leave the house. I experienced severe anxiety and panic attacks going shopping, and doing my evening job was sheer terror with the feeling of passing out, sickness and sweating. Fortunately, my husband took me to and picked me up from the school where I do two hours' cleaning. During the day when I had to go shopping, the feelings were so severe I used to wait for my children to come home from school then send them to do any shopping I needed.*

*However, after following your diet recommendations, the attacks lessened to such a degree I go out now without even thinking about it.*

*I started a new part-time office job. It started a day before my period was due and yet that week I didn't experience any problems at all. I went to town shopping after work, came home, cooked, cleaned, did my evening job and although I felt tired, at no time did I suffer from any feelings of panic or anxiety.*

*I went completely off the diet and ate and drank all the things I shouldn't have: within 48 hours I suffered really bad stomach ache and diarrhoea. All the feelings returned, so I am now back sticking strictly to your diet. Although I still have a queasy tum and headache, I can see myself getting back to normal.*

*The diet really works, I feel a new woman after six years of living in sheer hell.*

*Jane Moor*

### Dietary changes

*'I already knew I was allergic to eggs when I began the programme. It seems to run in my family. I was astonished, though, to be asked to give up all grains except brown rice, all sugar, tea and coffee and reduce my intake of dairy products.*

*I followed the diet rigidly for the first three months. I felt on top of the world. I lost weight, which was great, and was able to go out alone for the first time in six*

# PRE-MENSTRUAL SYNDROME QUESTIONNAIRE

Name: __Jane Moor_____  Age: __36____  Height: __5' 6"____  Weight: __11st 11lb__

MARITAL STATUS: Single_____ Married___✓___ Divorced_____ Widowed_____
(Please tick where applicable)

PRESENT CONTRACEPTION: None___✓___ Pill_____ I.U.D._____ Other_____

Your periods come every __26–30__ days     Your periods last ____4____ days

Your periods are: Light____✓____ Moderate_____ Heavy_____

Number of Pregnancies: ____3____     Number of Miscarriages:____–____

Birth weight of children: 1st Child_____ 2nd Child_____ 3rd Child_____ 4th Child_____

| SYMPTOMS | WEEK AFTER PERIOD (Fill in 3 days after period) | | | | WEEK BEFORE PERIOD (Fill in 2-3 days before period) | | | |
|---|---|---|---|---|---|---|---|---|
| | None | Mild | Moderate | Severe | None | Mild | Moderate | Severe |
| **PMT - A** | | | | | | | | |
| Nervous Tension | ✓ | | | | | | ✓ | |
| Mood Swings | ✓ | | | | | | ✓ | |
| Irritability | | ✓ | | | | | | ✓ |
| Anxiety | | | ✓ | | | | | ✓ |
| **PMT - H** | | | | | | | | |
| Weight gain | ✓ | | | | | | ✓ | |
| Swelling of Extremities | ✓ | | | | | ✓ | | |
| Breast Tenderness | ✓ | | | | | | | ✓ |
| Abdominal Bloating | ✓ | | | | | | | |
| **PMT - C** | | | | | | | | |
| Headache | | | ✓ | | | | | ✓ |
| Craving for Sweets | ✓ | | | | | ✓ | | |
| Increased Appetite | ✓ | | | | | ✓ | | |
| Heart Pounding | ✓ | | | | | | ✓ | |
| Fatigue | ✓ | | | | | | | ✓ |
| Dizziness or Fainting | | | ✓ | | | | ✓ | |
| **PMT - D** | | | | | | | | |
| Depression | ✓ | | | | | ✓ | | |
| Forgetfulness | ✓ | | | | | ✓ | | |
| Crying | ✓ | | | | | ✓ | | |
| Confusion | ✓ | | | | | ✓ | | |
| Insomnia | ✓ | | | | | | ✓ | |
| **OTHER SYMPTOMS** | | | | | | | | |
| Loss of Sexual Interest | | | ✓ | | | | ✓ | |
| Disorientation | ✓ | | | | | ✓ | | |
| Clumsiness | | | ✓ | | | | ✓ | |
| Tremors/Shakes | | ✓ | | | | ✓ | | |
| Thoughts of Suicide | ✓ | | | | | ✓ | | |
| Agoraphobia | | | ✓ | | | | | ✓ |
| Increased Physical Activity | ✓ | | | | | ✓ | | |
| Heavy/Aching Legs | ✓ | | | | | | ✓ | |
| Generalized Aches | ✓ | | | | | | ✓ | |
| Bad Breath | ✓ | | | | | ✓ | | |
| Sensitivity to Music/Light | ✓ | | | | | ✓ | | |
| Excessive Thirst | ✓ | | | | | ✓ | | |

# FOLLOW UP
## PRE-MENSTRUAL SYNDROME QUESTIONNAIRE

Name: __Jane Moor__          Age: __36__     Height: __5' 6"__     Weight: __11st 5lb__

MARITAL STATUS:     Single _____     Married __✓__     Divorced _____     Widowed _____
(Please tick where applicable)

PRESENT CONTRACEPTION:     None __✓__     Pill _____     I.U.D. _____     Other_____

    Your periods come every __26–30__ days     Your periods last __4__ days

    Your periods are:   Light ___✓___     Moderate _____     Heavy _____

SYMPTOMS

| | WEEK AFTER PERIOD (Fill in 3 days after period) | | | | WEEK BEFORE PERIOD (Fill in 2-3 days before period) | | | |
|---|---|---|---|---|---|---|---|---|
| | None | Mild | Moderate | Severe | None | Mild | Moderate | Severe |
| **PMT - A** | | | | | | | | |
| Nervous Tension | ✓ | | | | ✓ | | | |
| Mood Swings | ✓ | | | | ✓ | | | |
| Irritability | ✓ | | | | | ✓ | | |
| Anxiety | ✓ | | | | ✓ | | | |
| **PMT - H** | | | | | | | | |
| Weight gain | ✓ | | | | ✓ | | | |
| Swelling of Extremities | ✓ | | | | ✓ | | | |
| Breast Tenderness | ✓ | | | | | ✓ | | |
| Abdominal Bloating | ✓ | | | | | ✓ | | |
| **PMT - C** | | | | | | | | |
| Headache | ✓ | | | | ✓ | | | |
| Craving for Sweets | ✓ | | | | | ✓ | | |
| Increased Appetite | ✓ | | | | ✓ | | | |
| Heart Pounding | ✓ | | | | ✓ | | | |
| Fatigue | ✓ | | | | | ✓ | | |
| Dizziness or Fainting | ✓ | | | | ✓ | | | |
| **PMT - D** | | | | | | | | |
| Depression | ✓ | | | | ✓ | | | |
| Forgetfulness | ✓ | | | | ✓ | | | |
| Crying | ✓ | | | | ✓ | | | |
| Confusion | ✓ | | | | ✓ | | | |
| Insomnia | ✓ | | | | ✓ | | | |
| **OTHER SYMPTOMS** | | | | | | | | |
| Loss of Sexual Interest | ✓ | | | | ✓ | | | |
| Disorientation | ✓ | | | | ✓ | | | |
| Clumsiness | ✓ | | | | ✓ | | | |
| Tremors/Shakes | ✓ | | | | ✓ | | | |
| Thoughts of Suicide | ✓ | | | | ✓ | | | |
| Agoraphobia | ✓ | | | | | ✓ | | |
| Increased Physical Activity | ✓ | | | | | ✓ | | |
| Heavy/Aching Legs | ✓ | | | | | ✓ | | |
| Generalized Aches | ✓ | | | | | ✓ | | |
| Bad Breath | ✓ | | | | ✓ | | | |
| Sensitivity to Music/Light | ✓ | | | | ✓ | | | |
| Excessive Thirst | ✓ | | | | ✓ | | | |

*years. I got so much better that I am now able to hold down a full-time job. I have let the diet slip a bit more recently. You tend to take it all for granted when you are feeling really well. Plus it takes extra time and effort shopping for and preparing special food. I know that once I tighten my diet up again I will feel 100 per cent again.'*

All Jane's long-standing severe symptoms either cleared up completely or became very mild and 'livable' with. Diet was a major factor in her case, as she has proved to herself.

## CRIME OR ILLNESS?

Finally in this section, I return to the subject of violence. As violence in general is on the increase in our society I feel this is an area which is certainly worthy of fuller discussion.

As early as 1845 menstrually-related disorders were accepted by the courts as a defence for a criminal act. In that year there were three recorded examples:

- Martha, a servant who, without motive, murdered her employer's child, was acquitted on the grounds of insanity caused by 'obstructed menstruation'.

- A woman was acquitted of murdering her young niece on the grounds of insanity stemming from disordered menstruation.

- A woman servant was accused of theft and was acquitted at Carlisle quarter sessions on the grounds of temporary insanity 'from suppression of the menses'.

So you see, it's not such a new problem. We probably talk openly about it now, whereas years ago it would have been hushed up. More recently there have been other famous cases where PMT has been a large part of the defence.

Dr Dalton reported in *The Lancet* in 1980 the case of a 28-year-old worker in the food industry who was accused of fatally stabbing her girlfriend. Following the stabbing she was admitted to prison and noted to be menstruating. Although she was imprisoned, it was acknowledged that she had severe PMT which was subsequently treated. In 1982 she was freed on probation on the grounds of PMT.

There have been several other similar cases over the past few years. There was the case of Anna Reynolds who battered her mother to death in June 1986. She was convicted of murder in February 1987, and subsequently at appeal the charge was reduced to manslaughter on the basis of diminished responsibility whilst suffering with Pre-Menstrual Syndrome. Debra Lovell was another victim of PMT who became a human fireball after soaking herself in paraffin whilst she was pre-menstrual.

In November 1988 a teenage mother, Donna Kelly, suffering from PMT unintentionally killed her seven-week-old son by shaking him when he would not stop crying. The verdict recorded was not guilty as it was appreciated that Donna Kelly had previously been a loving mother who did not have the intention to kill her baby.

In May 1989 a mother of four killed her son after he 'wound her up'. She walked free from the Old Bailey after the judge said she was sick, rather than evil.

This evidence that some women become more vulnerable, unpredictable and even lose control pre-menstrually and around the time of the onset of their period, confirms the fact that the Pre-Menstrual Syndrome, or PMT to give it its other name, is a common condition which can be life-threatening and should most certainly be taken seriously.

It does, however, mean that PMT may be considered a plausible excuse for an offence. This, I am only too aware, is a very sensitive subject. Like any other scapegoat, it has and will, I'm sure, continue to be used in the courts as a means of reducing or escaping sentence.

Although, at the Women's Nutritional Advisory Service, we have encountered our share of criminal cases, I feel it is important to take a stand on this issue. There is no way that we condone any crime, or believe that a woman should be excused for her actions due to PMT. However, it is acknowledged that PMT can be a contributing factor which should be considered along with all the other factors in each individual case.

Each person, be they male or female, has the responsibility to look after their own body. There is evidence now, for example, that indicates that poor diet is related to delinquency and even dyslexia.

Rather than excusing women with PMT for their actions, or adolescents who offend for their behaviour, it would be better to help them overcome the problem by at least correcting their nutritional state. The upsetting and frustrating fact is that much education is needed, both for the public and also for the medical profession. Just knowing which foods help and which foods may harm would be a great start. Having some basic understanding of how diet can affect one's state of mind, for instance, would be invaluable.

We hope that over the next few years doctors will be taking all this into consideration, much more so than they are generally doing at present.

In the meantime, the courts have the difficult task of deciding where to draw the line. There should certainly be the facility for them to check on a woman's nutritional state and have her assessed for PMT. This assessment usually would take three months to confirm as three consecutive cycles need to be charted in order to confirm the diagnosis of PMT.

The fact that a woman may be a danger to herself or society has to be dealt with in a routine way by the courts. When PMT is presented as a defence or mitigation, and the diagnosis confirmed, then effective treatment should be sought whilst the woman is serving her sentence, if she has been convicted.

It is very important that when PMT is used as a defence or mitigation, appropriate treatment is instituted. It then becomes the woman's personal responsibility to follow the appropriate diet or take the appropriate treatment to ensure that her pre-menstrual symptoms are properly controlled. PMT could then not be used as a defence or mitigation should she then re-offend.

# 10

# THE SOCIAL
# IMPLICATIONS
# OF PMT

## RELATIONSHIPS AT HOME AND AT WORK

It was not surprising that as a result of these severe symptoms, we were recording that 95 per cent of our survey of women reported that their home lives and relationships with family and friends were affected by their PMT symptoms.

---

**Degree to which a sample
of 1000 women felt that their
home life/relationship with
family/friends was affected
due to PMT symptoms**

| Not Affected | Mild | Moderate | Severe | Total Affected |
|---|---|---|---|---|
| 4.9% | 12.7% | 36.1% | 46.3% - | 95.1% |

You will have read in earlier sections about how some family lives were affected. I have added two quite different examples here to make the point in its own right, as the family and our immediate circle are so very important.

Anita, who suffered severely with all four sub-groups, and actually attempted suicide, explains how she felt her home life was affected.

## ANITA'S PROBLEMS AT HOME

'From about 1982 I used to get so bad-tempered. I remember one day I was having an ordinary discussion with my husband and he made a comment which I took the wrong way. I started attacking him with a knife. Then I'd start attacking everybody else in the house except the baby, who I made a point of keeping away from.

I firmly believe that if we hadn't been having difficulties with our son at the time, my husband would have left me. I think he had got to the point where he couldn't take any more. My marriage was really under severe pressure. He was definitely on the point of saying "That's it".

I have two children and I think they have both been affected by my pre-menstrual behaviour. They learned to watch me carefully to see the mood I was in. This is because I would often attack them verbally and be cruel. Then afterwards I would pick them up and cuddle them. I couldn't always keep myself under control. They didn't understand. I think they have forgiven me now, but they still watch me. I don't think they can believe I'm not going to flip on them.'

Geraldine, whose worst problem was her secret chocolate binges, took her anger and frustration out on her daughters.

## GERALDINE'S FEELINGS OF ANGER

'I feel really aggressive towards the children, especially the older ones. I smack them in instances where it's not really deserved. I tend to take it out on the oldest daughter, even if she hasn't done anything to justify it.

The worst thing with the children is not so much the aggressiveness, because when I feel that way I try to keep away from them, but the sarcasm. I can be really horrible, and it's awful because it takes away all their self-confidence.

After being really awful I'd just go into the bedroom and lean my head on the wall and think, "Fancy saying something like that?" I'd feel really wicked and go into floods of tears. Sometimes I'd blame them and ask them how they could do this to me. I'd tell them that they were making me ill and accuse them of being horrid to me. Then I'd complain that they didn't do a thing around the house and threaten to get a maid. By this time they would be staring at me, absolutely rigid with fright. All the time, at the back of my mind I'd know I was being a bitch and feel crumby, really crumby because basically I love my girls to death and I don't want to say such awful things to them.'

92

## PRODUCTIVITY AND EFFICIENCY AT WORK

Another incredible statistic that emerged from the study on 1000 PMT sufferers was the degree to which their work suffered as a result of their symptoms. 92.7 per cent reported that their productivity and efficiency decreased pre-menstrually.

They further reported that they were, to a large degree, 'not there mentally' for an average of five days per month! This means that they produce very little work during this period of time.

A labour force survey conducted in 1985 found that there were just over ten million (10,104,000) working women between the ages of 16 and 44 in the UK. Just under seven million were employed and the remainder were self-employed. Given these figures the cost to industry due to lack of production must be vast, and probably not a statistic that has been properly considered. It wouldn't register as sickness or absenteeism as these women appear to be at work in the normal way. Unless specifically asked for, this information would not appear. Indeed, even asking for it may not produce the truth as there are so many women who would be in fear of losing their jobs. As it is, they feel they are teetering on the edge of disaster at work because of their general behaviour pre-menstrually. **81.6 per cent of 1000 women** felt that their work or career had been adversely affected by their PMT. So keeping a low profile is the least line of resistance.

---

**Effects on
productivity/efficiency
pre-menstrually out of
a sample of 1000 women**

---

| Same | Decreased | Increased |
|:---:|:---:|:---:|
| 6.2% | 92.7% | 1.1% |

---

A look at case histories of women who came to the Women's Nutritional Advisory Service proves the point. First there was Sally, a divorcee in an executive position.

## " Sally's Story "

'I have a very responsible, full-time position. My job involves dealing with people and quite a lot of travel. I found it very difficult to cope pre-menstrually. I felt emotionally unstable and frightened to go out of the house. It made me a liability, really. The moods I experienced gave me feelings of dislike for people I worked with for no apparent reason. Especially my manager.

I would be extremely bad-tempered and unable to concentrate. I had this persecution complex and felt that everybody was against me and scheming. If something went wrong I felt that it was other people's fault and that they were getting at me.

I would sometimes think "sod the lot of them, it's all their fault". I'd try to work, feeling so agitated and ill. I pushed myself to work even harder and faster, which made me even more tired and exhausted.'

Anita, a PMT D sufferer who had attempted suicide, had more than her share of problems at work.

## " Anita's Story "

'My work was certainly affected. I would forget things. Forget appointments and forget to put things in the diary. I just couldn't concentrate for that time of the month. In fact I was only normal for one week in four. For three weeks I'd feel so tired and work would take me much longer than usual. It would take me one to two hours to do half-an-hour's work. Consequently, for at least two weeks per month I'd have to work late to get my work done. Even then I'd still have to check all the work again when I wasn't pre-menstrual.'

## DRIVING ABILITY

Many of the symptoms discussed have broad repercussions on the sufferer herself and on her family and friends. However, the seriousness of PMT comes right home when a statistic appears that could affect us all. We asked 1000 drivers who suffer with PMT whether their driving ability was affected pre-menstrually. An astounding **76.9 per cent** said their driving ability decreased before their period. Many women stop driving pre-menstrually as they have previously had so many accidents pre-menstrually. The two main factors that seem to affect driving ability are lack of concentration and poor coordination. Amazingly, the women report that as soon as their period arrives, their driving ability returns to normal.

Driving a car, or any vehicle for that matter, is a real responsibility and not to be taken lightly. We advise severe sufferers to keep off the road until their symptoms have gone, or are under control. Placing lives at risk is no joke. Here are two examples of many who experienced diminished driving skills pre-menstrually.

## " Anita's Story "

'I have had several accidents and near-misses, all of which were during my pre-menstrual time. Once, when I was delivering a parcel, I went straight into the back of the car in front of me which was stationary. I didn't even see that he had stopped. Another time I was going to turn right, I saw something coming in the opposite direction and yet I carried on despite the fact that I'd seen the chap. I knew I hadn't got the speed to get past him, but I carried on nevertheless. I made lots of stupid decisions because I didn't have my mind on what was going on around me. I felt very vague and as if I was driving along in a metal box detached from reality. I have an excess on my insurance policy as a result of these accidents.'

## " Ruth's Story "

'If I was feeling aggressive generally pre-menstrually, then I would be aggressive behind the wheel. I can remember once, there was a stupid man in a van in front of me at a junction. He was over the white line on the middle of the road. He was going right and I was going left, I was feeling all steamed up. I was alone in the car. I mounted the pavement to get past him, revving up hard and hooting the horn. In fact I scraped my car all along his mudguard. Then I zoomed off. That was typical of how I used to feel. I have still got the car with the mark.'

# 11

# WHY IS PMT
# MORE COMMON
# TODAY?

I am forever being asked the question 'Why is PMT more common these days?' In order to understand why, we need to take a look at twentieth-century diet and lifestyle. In reality, it is not just PMT which seems to be affecting more women nowadays, but a whole gamut of medical conditions. In many cases the conditions are diet-related. I don't expect you really to believe such a statement at this point in time. Bear with me, and allow me to present some facts. There are some shocks and surprises in store – BEWARE!

In Great Britain it is thought that more than 150,000 people die every year from heart attacks and strokes. Thirty-five million Americans now suffer with high blood pressure, which is no doubt a contributory factor to the one and a half million heart attacks and strokes that occur each year. Ill health is costing the taxpayer a fortune, literally. It is estimated that in the UK it costs the taxpayer at least £12,000 million per year, some three times more than in 1949. In the USA in the last 20 or so years the medical bill has increased from $27 billion to $200 billion! The awful fact is that, despite these amounts of money being spent, some of us have been getting sicker.

'Mental' illness is on the increase, hyperactivity in children is not uncommon, and allergies such as eczema, asthma and hay fever are increasingly common. As we age, those of us who don't get cancer seem to get arthritis or diabetes. It appears that we are being crippled slowly and subtly. Although real advances have been made in the treatment of kidney disease and diabetes and in heart surgery, it is prevention, rather than new treatments, that is now needed.

In 1986 the Women's Nutritional Advisory Service completed a national street survey on 500 women in Britain. We found that 73.6 per cent of them suffered in varying degrees with PMT. This figure is considerably more than estimates of 30–60 per cent made during the previous 30 years.

By now you must be wondering why the diseases are becoming more common, and you might well ask. Our twentieth-century lifestyle brings many relatively new experiences to us, some of which we are not well equipped to handle. The diets most of us know are very far removed from that of our ancestors. Our bodies were not built to cope with refined and processed foods, very often empty of nutrients. We have had to live with pesticides and insecticides being sprayed on our crops, growth hormones and antibiotics pumped into animals, and environmental pollution and acid rain as the finishing touches. Many of us over-eat and under-exercise, and women nowadays tend to lead far more stressful existences. So it is logical, really, that we can't honestly expect our 'machines' to go on indefinitely without breaking down when we don't treat them with respect. We generally treat our cars better than we do our bodies – you wouldn't dream of putting the wrong fuel in your petrol tank, would you?

Before I launch into the tale of woe about our diet, let me say that although you will probably come to realize that we are faced with certain problems concerning our diet, with good education we *can* find ways around them. I will of course be discussing various solutions in the Self-Help section on diet in Part Three.

## A GOOD LOOK AT OUR DIET

In order to look at diet more closely we need to examine how our habits have changed during this century.

- We have increased our consumption of sugar. The UK has become one of the world's largest sweet eaters, consuming 75 lb or 37 kilos of sugar per person per year.

- Our diet is particularly high in saturated fats (animal fats). It is thought that this has much to do with our also having a high incidence of heart disease and breast cancer.

- We eat far too much salt – 10 to 20 times more than our bodies really require per day. Salt can contribute to blood pressure problems and pre-menstrual water retention.

- We often drink far too much coffee and tea which block the absorption of essential nutrients. On average we consume four cups of tea and two cups of coffee per day, but many people exceed this.

- We consume volumes of foods with a high level of phosphorus, which impedes absorption of good nutrients. Examples of these foods are soft drinks and low or normal calorie types of processed foods, canned, packaged, pre-packed, convenience foods and ready-made sauces.

- Many of the foods available contain chemical additives in the form of flavour enhancers, colouring and preservatives. Whilst some of these are not harmful, some of them *are*, and our bodies are certainly not designed to cope with them.

- Our water contains certain pollutants which are thought to be a risk to public health.

- Our meat has become contaminated with antibiotics and growth hormones.

- Nitrate fertilizers have been used to obtain fast-growing and abundant crops. It is now recognized that nitrates are harmful and can produce cancer, at least in animals.

- Almost all of our fresh fruit, cereals and vegetables are sprayed with pesticides at least once. In addition, milk and meat may retain the pesticides from feed given to livestock.

### Smoking

Smoking tobacco has become a widespread habit among Western societies. In 1922 in the United Kingdom, for example, 20–34-year-old women smoked an average of fifty cigarettes per year, but by 1975 this had risen to an average of just over three thousand cigarettes per woman, per year. Despite the more educated classes reducing their cigarette consumption, smoking has become relatively more common amongst women, in those who are less well educated.

### Alcohol

Since the 1940s alcohol consumption has doubled in the United Kingdom. On average, women consume one unit of alcohol per day, and men three units (one unit = 1 glass of wine, 1 pub measure of spirits, 1 small sherry or vermouth, or half a pint of normal strength beer or lager). These average levels are now the maximum recommended daily intakes for women and men respectively. Whilst many of us may be teetotallers, or drink substantially less than this, there will be those who regularly consume more. Some women may go on pre-menstrual alcohol binges.

For every £1 spent on food in the United Kingdom, some 75p is spent on alcohol and tobacco. Just think how the quality of the food in the United Kingdom could improve if only half the money spent on alcohol and tobacco was spent on purchasing better quality food.

## Drugs

Western societies have become drug-oriented. In the USA in 1984 over $2000 billion was spent on drugs. In 1983, according to the Institute for the Study of Drug Dependence, £1600 million was spent on drugs, 50 per cent more than was spent in 1980. In the UK, over £40 million per year is spent on tranquillizers alone, with approximately 32 million prescriptions being written for them, many of which are repeat prescriptions.

In the last year there has been tremendous concern by medical practitioners worldwide about the excessive use of benzodiazepene tranquillizers and sleeping tablets. It is now recommended that these drugs, which include Valium, Mogadon and Ativan, are used as a temporary measure for only a few weeks. Those who have been taking them long-term should, if at all possible, have their dosage and frequency gradually reduced under medical supervision.

## The Pill

The oral contraceptive birth control pill has been a popular and effective method of contraception. The initial forms of the oral contraceptive pill had high levels of oestrogen, which were known to cause some disturbance in vitamin and mineral balance, increase the risk of vaginal thrush, and in some women precipitate significant depression and migraine headaches. These side-effects are less likely with the new lower dose, or phased dosage oral contraceptive pill. However, problems can certainly arise. Whilst the oral contraceptive pill can help some women's pre-menstrual symptoms, and is a useful way for treating mild PMT, particularly in those women who require contraception, it can also aggravate some PMT symptoms. There is no way of determining this, other than by trial and error. If you find an oral contraceptive pill that suits you, all well and good. However, some women will find that practically any form of the Pill aggravates their pre-menstrual symptoms.

## Vitamin and mineral intake

Our diet this century has gone through, and continues to go through, several substantial changes. By the end of the 1970s there was evidence, from certain surveys, of a deterioration in the quality of the UK diet, particularly since the Second World War. A high intake of sugar, refined foods, animal fats and alcohol had meant a relatively poor intake of essential vitamins and minerals.

Some fifteen vitamins, twenty-four minerals and eight amino acids have been isolated as being essential for normal body function. They are synergistic, which means that they rely upon each other in order to keep the body functioning at an optimum level. When one or more is in short supply, alterations in body metabolism occur. Minor deficiencies can often be tolerated, but major or multiple deficiencies result in the body becoming inefficient, with the development of symptoms and possibly disease.

There is, however, some heartening recent evidence. All the good advice from numerous individual experts and expert committees, government ones included, has finally got through to the British public. We have begun to cut down our intake of saturated animal fats, and increased our consumption of fibre from wholegrains, fruit and vegetables. The intake of sugar has also been falling in some sectors of the population. The main stimulus for concern about diet in the UK has been our relatively high rate of heart disease. The types of dietary changes above may not only prove to be helpful to reduce heart disease risk, but may also reduce the future risk of developing cancer, and other more immediate conditions, such as PMT.

Let us now turn our attention to certain specific nutrients which may contribute to symptoms of PMT.

## THE NITTY GRITTY
## REVIEW OF SPECIFIC NUTRIENTS

Some nutritional factors may be of particular importance to PMT. In the United Kingdom, the Department of Health has instructed the Committee on the Medical Aspects of Food to investigate the nature of the UK diet, and what the appropriate intakes of calories, fats, fibre, vitamins and minerals should be. A similar governmental review by the Food and Drug Administration in the USA was also undertaken in the mid-1980s, but without any final agreement being made.

Hopefully, new, up-to-date figures for Recommended Daily Allowances for essential nutrients in both the UK and US will be set, and we'll be better able to judge how our current diets achieve this, and what dietary changes we, as a nation, should make.

### Vitamin B

The B group of vitamins, and in particular vitamin B6, have been used for many years to treat PMT. In the UK there is no Recommended Daily Allowance (RDA) for vitamin B6, but in the US that is 2 mg per person per day. In 1956, vitamin B6 contained in the British Household Food Supply (food eaten in the home), was 1.6 to 1.9 mg per person per day. By 1976 this had dropped to 1.3 mg per person per day, but the most recent figures for 1986 show a rise to 1.91 mg.

However, in 1985 the Booker Health Report revealed in its independent study that the average intake for females was 1.2 mg per day. Other studies have shown that laboratory evidence of vitamin B6 deficiency from blood tests is a common finding in subjects with anxiety and depression, and even 15 per cent of the healthy, well-fed female population may have evidence of deficiency.

Many refined foods are low in B complex vitamins. For example, a McDonald's Big Mac hamburger is known to contain only a fraction of the vitamin B6 that it should do. Presumably, substantial quantities are lost in preparation, cooking and storage. In fact, you would have to eat sixty Big Mac hamburgers a day, in order to achieve an intake of 1.2 mg of vitamin B6 – a current conservative Recommended Daily Allowance.

Thus, for some of us whose diets do not contain good quantities of fresh and wholesome foods, the intake of B vitamins, and in particular vitamin B6, may be low.

### Magnesium

Magnesium is a key mineral in the treatment of PMT. It has now been shown in three medical studies that women with PMT have low levels of magnesium in their red blood cells.

Once again, there is no UK RDA for magnesium; in the USA the RDA range is between 300–450 mg per person per day: it seems to vary from state to state.

According to a report entitled 'Nutrients in the United States Food Supply, 1909–1965', the decreased use of grain products is the primary reason for the magnesium deficiency. In 1909 grains furnished some 37 per cent of the total magnesium intake in the USA, compared with only 18 per cent in 1965.

Magnesium content of the average British housewife's diet is barely adequate, at 249 mg per day. Many will be below this, and at risk of deficiency, especially if consuming alcoholic drinks, soft drinks or large quantities of refined carbohydrates and sugar. The latest figures for 1986 suggest a small rise in magnesium intake in the British diet, but still below that of the UK Recommended Daily Allowance.

### Iron

It is probably better known that menstruating women have an increased need for the mineral iron; in fact, iron levels are at their lowest four days pre-menstrually. This time there *is* an RDA in the UK for iron, which is 12 mg per day; this is somewhat lower than the RDA for the USA, which is 18 mg.

The Booker Health Report showed that 60 per cent of females between the ages of 18 and 54 have iron levels below the recommended daily allowance. In another study in 1984, it was found that a group of 15–25-year-old women consumed only 75 per cent of the RDA for iron, so many are at risk of deficiency.

Consuming a cup of tea with a meal will reduce the absorption of iron from all non-animal foods in the diet.

### Zinc and other trace minerals

Zinc and trace minerals, such as copper, chromium and selenium, do not have RDA values set for the UK at present. Our intakes, like iron, are probably adequate if one eats a healthy, well-balanced diet. The refining and processing of foods reduces their trace nutrient content substantially. There is no evidence that there are substantial deficiencies of these in the general population, if they are eating well. However, for those of us who rely upon convenience foods, or simply do not have the funds for a well-balanced healthy diet, intake can be poor. Meat, fresh vegetables, nuts, seeds, and other wholefoods are good sources of these trace minerals, but are relatively expensive to buy when compared with sugar, margarine and white bread. In the 1986 Booker Health Report, 70 per cent of the sample of women aged between 18 and 54 had a dietary intake of zinc below the World Health Organization recommended level of 11 mg. This is confirmed by an average intake in the 1986 British Household Food Supply of 9 mg per day.

## IT'S A POOR SHOW

It seems astonishing to consider that such important nutrients are acknowledged to be in such short supply, and yet not a great deal is being done to reverse the trend. Three out of four of these nutrients do not even have a Recommended Daily Allowance in the UK.

When you read the section on Vitamins and Minerals in Chapter 13, pay particular attention to these four important nutrients, notice what their function is in the body and what happens to us if we don't get them in sufficient quantities. Is it any wonder that our bodies are slowly going to seed when we are not providing them with the essential materials they need in order for them to function properly?

In the Self-Help section, I concentrate on foods that contain a high level of these particular nutrients as well as a few others. I will help you to work out a diet for yourself which will provide you with good amounts of the essential nutrients that you are most likely to be short of.

### Other barriers

Not only may we be taking in insufficient amounts of vitamins and minerals, but the value of many of these nutrients is impaired by factors like alcohol, tea, coffee and tobacco.

Another thing to bear in mind which severely lowers the nutritional value of food is the cooking process. For example, boiling a cabbage rids it of about 75 per cent of its vitamin C. Baking or frying food can destroy up to 50 per cent of other vitamins. Commercially frozen vegetables can also be lacking in some nutrients by as much as 47 per cent though usually they are the next best thing to fresh ones, since canning can result in up to 70 per cent of the nutritional content being lost. It appears that processing food does little to enhance our health at the end of the day.

A good example of the effect of processing on nutrient content, is the nutrient content of some of McDonald's foods. I am sorry to keep using them as an example, but at least they are one of the few fast-food manufacturers who have had the nerve to assess the nutrient content of their own products. A McDonald's apple pie in fact contains no vitamin C whatsoever, according to their own analysis. It should contain several milligrams, and presumably it has been lost by excessive cooking of the apples. Other commercial apple pies may not be any better.

By now you no doubt realize that a 'normal healthy diet' is somewhat of a myth. Although it is possible to eat a nutritious diet, you need to be fairly educated on the subject before you can even make a start. Then, as you can see, there are numerous hurdles to be overcome.

Whilst all these facts do seem depressing, there is a light at the end of the tunnel. In the Self-Help section on diet I will be concentrating on which types of foods to buy, and suggesting methods of preparation that will preserve the nutrients in your food.

## TIMES DO CHANGE

Is it any wonder women suffer with PMT! One hundred years ago, meat, animal fat and sugar were a much smaller part of our diets than today. The consumption of cereal fibres has also dropped by as much as 90 per cent. These are important factors in relation to PMT, as you will see.

It has become far more difficult to eat a 'normal healthy diet'. However, if you concentrate on avoiding the nutrient-deficient and contaminated foods listed below, you will be making changes for the better in your diet, which will not only help your PMT, but will help you feel healthier all round. There is less you can do to combat the unhealthy effects of the polluted environment, but I make some suggestions below.

**The diet of our ancestors.** When we examine the diet of our ancestors, we then begin to realize that it is not 'natural' to eat meat in the quantity that the majority of us do today. Evidence shows that diet approximately three million years ago consisted largely of hard seeds, plant fibre, some roots and stems – a diet high in vegetable matter similar to that of the Guinea baboon today.

103

Animals today are bred to be fat. Modern meat contains some seven times more fat than the wild meat our ancestors ate. Our ancestors' meat also contained five times more of the good polyunsaturated fats than today's meat, which is high in the potentially harmful saturated fats. The ancient diet was also richer in vitamins and minerals and polyunsaturated fats, and many times richer than the modern diet. It was a diet which was largely composed of fresh raw foods.

**Antibiotics.** Because antibiotics are being so widely used on animals, the conditions that would normally be treated by antibiotics are becoming resistant to them. Apart from being used as a medicine for individual sick animals, they are given to whole herds as a preventive measure, and they are again used for growth promotion.

My advice is to try to use organic or additive-free meat where possible, meat which has not been subjected to drugs, growth promoters or contaminated foods. Organic and additive-free meat is becoming more and more available. Certainly local farms and even supermarkets often keep stocks. If you can find 'clean' meat, it can be included in your diet approximately three times per week. An alternative is to limit one's meat intake to moderate quantities of good-quality lean meat, or to become a vegetarian. It's the fat in the meat that will carry much of the pollutants, so avoid it – and also rely more on fish. When eating chicken, don't eat the skin and don't make the gravy from the fatty part of the juices, pour it off first.

**Fat consumption.** Britain has the honour of having the highest incidence of heart disease in the world. This was not so in the past, when other countries such as Finland and Australia were way ahead. Something drastic must have happened to change statistics so dramatically.

It seems that the saturated fats increase the level of cholesterol which leaves the bloodstream and settles down in the arteries, resulting in a gradual blockage of those supplying the heart, brain and other organs. This leads to heart attacks, strokes and poor circulation. Smoking accelerates the process.

By 1966 the Australian and US rate of heart disease began to decline, but that was not so for Britain, whose casualties were on the increase.

In other countries such as Finland, for example, who were previously 'top of the coronary pops', a national nutritional education campaign was undertaken. The result now is that they are a much healthier nation with a far lower incidence of heart disease than many other countries.

**The sweet facts.** Over the past 100 years there has been a 25-fold increase in world sugar production. This is a real change from the days when sugar was an expensive luxury that we locked away for high days and holidays, and was only consumed at all by the wealthy. Refined sugars simply didn't exist for our ancestors. Their diet consisted mainly of vegetables, fruit, cereals and some wild meat. It wasn't until this century that we developed an addiction to the sweet and sticky sugar family.

We clearly don't need refined sugar. What seems to have been overlooked is that our bodies can change complex carbohydrates and proteins into the sugar they require. Sugar contains no vitamins, no minerals, no protein, no fibre, no starches. It may contain tiny traces of calcium and magnesium if you're lucky, and it certainly provides us with loads of calories (kjs), 'empty calories'.

It is actually a fair skill these days not to consume large amounts of sugar, because it is added to so many foods. What do you think the following have in common? Cheese, biscuits, fruit yogurt, tomato sauce, baked beans, pickled cucumbers, muesli, beefburgers, Worcester sauce, pork sausages, peas, cornflakes and Coca-Cola – well, they can all contain sugar. Coca-Cola contains some seven teaspoonfuls per can.

There are some more nutritious alternatives which I will discuss in the Self-Help section. The food manufacturers are beginning to understand that their consumers are waking up, and the majority actually don't want to be dumped on. For now my advice is to read the labels carefully when you are shopping: I guarantee you will have a few surprises!

### Water

Our most important nutrient is water, and sadly it is becoming one of our major sources of pollution. Not only is the water contaminated with lead, aluminium and copper, we now have nitrates to contend with as well. Nitrates are chemicals used in fertilizers to promote crop growth.

**Why are nitrates harmful?** Well, they go through chemical changes and at the end of the day turn into nitrosamines which are believed to be strong cancer-producing chemicals. They also block the absorption of essential nutrients, which are necessary for the resolution of PMT symptoms.

### Toxic minerals

Toxic minerals in the form of lead, mercury and copper are in the soil, the air and the water, as well as being present in our food. During this century their levels have been rising rapidly, and at times to a point where our bodies have not been able to cope.

**Lead.** Lead pollution has been much discussed in the media over the past few years. High lead levels are acknowledged to be linked to low birth weight and low intelligence in children. As a result of extensive research on lead, many countries have removed lead from petrol and are trying to keep lead levels down in cities. However, it is far more difficult to remove it from the water supply as the filtering systems at water purification plants can't cope with the load.

**Copper.** Although copper is an essential mineral, in excess it can be pretty damaging. In fact, an excess of copper may be linked to miscarriages, premature babies, post-natal depression and mental illnesses.

We are exposed to copper in our everyday lives without realizing it. There are water pipes that contain copper, some kitchen utensils, jewellery, IUD – copper coils – and even the anti-fungal agents at the swimming pool usually contain copper.

Our daily requirement of copper is about 2 mg, most of which is obtained from water and food.

It's worth bearing in mind that copper cancels out zinc. For every one part of copper, 14 parts of zinc are needed to balance it. Make sure from the container that this ratio exists in the supplements you buy: you'll be surprised to find that in many cases it doesn't.

## Helpful tips to avoid the TOXINS

- Concentrate on eating a nutritious diet, particularly high in zinc, magnesium, calcium and vitamins C and B.

- Take a well-balanced multi-vitamin supplement and some extra vitamin C if you are at particular risk.

- Scrub all fruit and vegetables with a brush to clean off as many toxins as possible, and remove the outer layers of lettuce and cabbage, etc. Don't peel fruit and vegetables unless you don't like the peel – very often the bulk of the nutrients is just under the skin. Use organic vegetables and salad stuff or grow your own where possible, without using chemicals.

- Water filters tend to filter out a good deal of the toxic metals. Water purifiers can be bought in healthfood shops, but they aren't so efficient. Every so often the filter needs replacing – and it's amazing what collects in it. Rather the toxic deposits collect in the filter than your body!

## Avoid:

- Spending too much time near busy roads if the local exhaust fumes contain lead (which may be easier said than done).

- Copper and aluminium cookware unless with a non-stick lining.

- Alcohol, as it increases lead absorption.

- Refined foods which give the body little protection against toxins.

- Antacids which contain aluminium salts.

### Food additives

Whilst, of course, there are some perfectly harmless substances added to food, the number of potentially harmful additives is significant. Many additives have been shown to cause hyperactivity in children, asthma, eczema, skin rashes and swelling. It's obviously important to be able to differentiate between the safe and not-so-safe additives.

After being bombarded by warnings about additives is it any wonder that some of us have at one time or another avoided all foods containing them? Understandably, 'additive' has become a dirty word in some circles. But it's important to understand that some additives are, in fact, beneficial! For example: beneficial additives include riboflavin – vitamin B2 – and calcium L-Ascorbate which is vitamin C, and the many preservatives which help keep our food from spoiling.

## WHICH ADDITIVES ARE SAFE?

Fortunately, there is now no need to remain confused about which additives are safe and which are potentially harmful. Look in Appendix 2 on p 224 for details of booklets and books on additives which will help you to pick out the dangerous additives from the safe ones.

### Coffee

Over the last 10 years reports have begun to filter through about the health hazards attached to coffee consumption. Probably one of the reasons why these facts are now coming to light is that increasing amounts of coffee are being consumed. Since 1950 the consumption of coffee in the UK has increased fourfold and according to the US Department of Agriculture, in 1984 10.4 lb (4.6 kg) of coffee were consumed per person in the USA. Many people become quite addicted to it unknowingly, and couldn't give up the habit easily.

We now know that coffee worsens pre-menstrual breast tenderness, aggravates nervous tension, anxiety and insomnia and is even thought to be linked to heart disease! So obviously, no matter how much we may enjoy it, drinking coffee to excess is not a healthy habit. In fact, coffee contains caffeine which is a mental and physical stimulant. This can be of benefit of course, but even with 2–4 cups per day, adverse effects can be experienced. These include anxiety, restlessness, nervousness, insomnia, rapid pulse, palpitations, shakes and passing increased quantities of water. Regular coffee drinkers not only enjoy the flavour, but in many cases come to rely on the stimulation to get them through the day. If you cannot get going without your first fix of the day, you know what I mean!

Weaning yourself off coffee can sometimes be a fairly traumatic experience. It can sometimes produce symptoms not unlike a drug withdrawal, in particular a severe headache, which may take several days to disappear. However, rest assured they do eventually go completely, as long as you manage to abstain from coffee.

### Ways to go about giving up coffee

- Cut down gradually over the space of a week or two.

- Use decaffeinated coffee instead of coffee containing caffeine, but limit yourself to 2–3 cups per day.

- Try alternative drinks like Barleycup or Bambu which you can obtain from healthfood shops.

- If you like filter coffee, you can still use your filter, but with decaffeinated versions or with roasted dandelion root instead of coffee. You can obtain dried roasted dandelion root from good healthfood shops. It may sound a bit way out, but it has a very pleasant malted flavour.

**Decaffeinated coffee.** The bad news is not completely over! Coffee also contains other chemicals such as methylxanthines, which have been associated with cancer and premature ageing. So decaffeinated coffee as a substitute should still be kept to moderate levels.

If you continue to drink small amounts of coffee, it's best not to drink it at mealtimes. Research indicates that the absorption of zinc and iron from food decreases if coffee is consumed with a meal. These two are important minerals, particularly to PMT sufferers.

### Tea

The British are famous for their tea consumption. Tea, like coffee, contains caffeine, about 50 mg per cup, compared to coffee's 100 mg per strong cup. Tea also contains tannin, which inhibits the absorption of zinc and iron in particular. Excess tea produces the same effects as coffee, and you can also experience a withdrawal headache. Tea can also cause constipation.

By drinking a cup of tea with a meal you can cut down the absorption of iron from vegetarian foods to one-third. Whereas, a glass of fresh orange juice with the same meal would increase iron absorption by two times because of its high vitamin C content. Vegetarian and vegan women need their intake of iron to be readily absorbed. Therefore, drinking anything other than small amounts of weak tea may mean they risk becoming iron deficient.

'Herbal teas' don't count as tea as such. It's really a confusing name. Most herbal teas are free of caffeine and tannin and just consist of a collection of herbs. Unlike regular tea, they can be cleansing and relaxing.

## Alcohol

Alcohol is causing far greater problems to our society than most of us realize. It is the drug most seriously abused. Young people tend to begin drinking at an earlier age than was the case in previous generations. Public attitudes to drinking have become much more liberal and gradually alcohol has become widely socially accepted, without an appreciation of its adverse effects.

A major factor explaining the rise in alcohol consumption appears to be the decline in the real price of alcohol. It's not alcohol itself that has gone down in price, but the amount of work necessary to earn the cost of a drink.

Before I go any further I must state that I am not addressing alcoholics as such in this section but 'social drinkers'; those who like to have a few drinks, two or three times a week, can be jeopardizing their health. Anything above the national average for women, that is one glass of wine or half a pint of beer or one sherry or vermouth per day, means running some degree of health risk. Men consume on average three times this amount, and are recommended to halve it.

Alcohol in excess destroys body tissue over the years, and can cause or contribute to many diseases. For example, cardiovascular diseases, digestive disorders, inflammation and ulceration of the lining of the digestive tract, liver disease, brain degeneration, miscarriages, damage to unborn children and malnutrition, are some of the conditions associated with the long-term use of alcohol. In particular, certain vitamins and minerals are destroyed or lost from the body, including vitamin B1, thiamin, magnesium, zinc, vitamin B6, pyridoxine, calcium and vitamin D. All of these nutrients are particularly important to PMT sufferers, as you will see in Chapter 13.

As most of these conditions come on gradually, we often don't see the real dangers of alcohol. There is no impact like that of an accident, or the drama of an ambulance arriving to carry you off. But instead, there is a slow process of destruction which conveniently escapes our awareness.

Amongst those PMT sufferers who like a regular drink are those who increase their consumption considerably before their period. If this happens to you, then you will be well aware of the social problems that go with it, such as mood swings and personality changes. When this occurs others around become affected, and relationships may be strained at home and at work. It is a fact that one-third of the divorce petitions cite alcohol as a contributory factor and one-third of child abuse cases are linked to heavy drinking by a parent. Local courtrooms are always having to deal with people who committed offences whilst under the influence of alcohol. Offences that might never have been committed, were it not for that 'one for the road'!

### Old habits die hard

The type of food you eat is usually determined by you. However, there are many other factors that influence your 'preferences' through your life. The two main influential factors are:

1   Your parents, who introduce you to your initial diet, based on their preferences and their knowledge about diet.

The chances are that you continue to eat many of the foods introduced to you by your parents through your life. Habit patterns are quite hard to change, and a very important factor, of course, is that you've got to want to change them.

2   The exposure to the media which we all have in the form of advertisements on television, in magazines, billboards, etc. Now, the second factor, the power or persuasion via the media, might be highly desirable – if it was good food that was being promoted. If the media were dedicated to educating the public about a good, wholesome, nutritious diet, a more valuable asset we could not wish for! In reality they are there to persuade us, on behalf of the food industry, that fast foods, processed foods, or convenience foods, call them what you will, are desirable. They would have us believe that coffee is relaxing and that we should switch to cola-based drinks.

Rather than being a help educationally, they are often a great hindrance. Considering how much television we watch, is it any wonder that the hypnotic powers of the media begin to affect many of us, who would otherwise be influenced by common sense and our own good judgement?

### Take one positive step at a time

I am sorry to bombard you with so many depressing facts all at once. We the consumers definitely need more information about the food we eat and the environmental factors we are subjected to.

Probably the first step towards reversing the effects of the twentieth century on your body is for you to acknowledge the value of that body if you haven't already done so. After all, we only have one body to last us through a lifetime, so it's important to treat it with respect.

It's up to you how often you expose your body to alcohol, cigarettes, drugs and additives, and how physically fit you keep through exercise. Making one change at a time is better than not changing at all. I will be concentrating on how to go about making changes in the Self-Help section of the book, Part Three.

As for environmental pollution, there are now many worthwhile national and local groups running campaigns to help overcome these problems. You will find a list of these in Part Four. If you are concerned about your local situation, you can always contact the government representative for your area for help and advice.

If you have been neglecting your body to some extent, now may be the time to take stock. Don't expect your doctor to piece you back together again when you have fallen apart through 'environmental wear and nutritional tear'!

It's up to each one of us to look after our bodies to the best of our abilities and to treat them as well as any other of our treasured possessions.

# 12

# A REVIEW OF NUTRITIONAL, DRUG AND HORMONAL TREATMENTS

## INTRODUCTION

Many different treatments have been tried for Pre-Menstrual Syndrome or PMT. The wide variety of different treatments would itself suggest that no one single treatment is universally successful, and this indeed is the case. In fact, the greatest difficulty is finding out which treatment is suitable for which sufferers.

There are advantages and disadvantages to all forms of treatment. The type of treatment should also match the level of symptoms. Mild symptoms might be treated by a few simple changes in diet, or supplements of vitamin B6. The more severely affected sufferer, who is driven to distraction at the expense of her personal and family life, may require very strict dietary treatment, the use of high doses of certain vitamins and minerals, or some of the more established hormonal treatments.

On the whole, the majority of us would want to select a treatment that is effective, free from side effects, easy to administer and produces lasting benefit. The nutritional approach will therefore often be appropriate. Treatment with drugs, hormones and even nutritional supplements may not always produce lasting benefit, so attention to diet and lifestyle is almost always appropriate.

## TYPES OF TREATMENT

The types of treatment can be broadly divided into the following:

**Nutritional Supplements:** These include vitamin B6, multi-vitamins, with high dose vitamin B6 and magnesium, e.g. Optivite, evening primrose oil, e.g. Efamol, and vitamin E.

**Dietary treatment:** As already detailed, improving the quality of diet by reducing the intake of social poisons and increasing nutrient quality, is a common approach.

**Drug therapies:** Several different drugs have been used, including pain killers, diuretics, antidepressants and sedatives. They may each affect individual PMT symptoms, but do not usually address the cause.

**Hormonal treatments:** These include natural progesterone, synthetic progesterone, the oral contraceptive pill, oestrogen implants and other drugs with hormone-like activity.

On the whole, drug and hormonal treatments can, if they are effective, work very quickly. Dietary change, unless adhered to very strictly, may take two or three months to be effective, and the same seems to be true of vitamin preparations. At times it may be appropriate for some women to take a drug or hormonal therapy in the short term whilst a nutritional approach is also being tried to produce a more lasting benefit.

For some women there will be no choice but to try a variety of different therapies under the guidance of their GP or specialist. Even whilst this is occurring there is no reason why you can't take measures to try to help yourself by attention to diet, lifestyle and exercise.

On the whole, in the last ten years, there has been a shying away from over-reliance upon drug-based therapies, both by the public and medical profession. The shadow cast by the excessive use of benzodiazepene tranquillizers has yet to be fully dispelled from UK prescribing habits. This has resulted in a significant loss of confidence by the public in the 'pill for every ill' philosophy.

So let us look at the different treatments in more detail.

## Nutritional Supplements:

**Vitamin B6** – pyridoxine – was first tried in the treatment of Pre-Menstrual Tension back in 1972. Since then eleven properly conducted studies have been performed and published in a variety of medical journals. Not all showed a beneficial effect of pyridoxine. On the whole, a mild to moderate beneficial effect from pyridoxine can be achieved with dosages between 50 and 200 mg per day, taken throughout the menstrual cycle. Dosages less than 50 mg may not be effective. If no benefit is observed after two to three months, then a different treatment should be tried.

A multi-vitamin/multi-mineral preparation which contains high doses of vitamin B6, other B complex vitamins, magnesium and other minerals has been used in the treatment of PMT. This preparation, Optivite, has, in three out of four properly conducted studies, shown a beneficial effect. The dosage recommended is in the region of four to six tablets a day, which would provide 200–300 mg of vitamin B6. Vitamin B6 requires other B complex vitamins and magnesium in order to be converted into its active form.

**Evening primrose oil:** Six studies on evening primrose oil, Efamol, have shown a beneficial effect. However, in some studies the benefit was mild, or limited only to a few types of symptoms, e.g. depression. Evening primrose oil seems to be particularly helpful for benign breast disease, including pre-menstrual breast tenderness. The effective dosage is between six and eight 500 mg capsules per day throughout the cycle. This makes it a costly treatment.

**Vitamin E:** One study has demonstrated the effectiveness, at a dosage of 150–600 IU per day throughout the cycle. Anxiety and depressive symptoms seem to be helped in particular.

Side-effects of nutritional products are rare. There have been reports of vitamin B6, pyridoxine, producing nerve damage, which caused symptoms of numbness, tingling and pain in the arms and legs. This has occurred with dosages of 500 mg per day or more. Reports of such have been practically confined to the United States, and no confirmed reports have occurred in the United Kingdom. We consider dosages of up to 200 mg a day of pyridoxine to be safe. Higher doses, when taken in conjunction with other B vitamins and minerals, may also be safe. In particular, to the best of our knowledge at the time of printing, no reports of nerve damage have occurred in subjects taking Optivite, even in very large doses. Evening primrose oil has few side-effects, but it should not be administered to those who have epilepsy.

Vitamin E at dosages of up to 600 IU a day is practically harmless, unless the subject is also on anticoagulants – blood-thinning drugs.

### Dietary Treatments:

In 1988 the leading medical journal, *The Lancet*, carried a report by Dr Boyd and colleagues from the United States. They studied the effects of dietary change in women with benign breast disease who experienced pre-menstrual breast tenderness. They compared the effect of consuming an average US diet – similar to that

114

of the UK, with a low fat, high complex-carbohydrate diet. The reduction in fats was mainly from saturated fats, and the increase in complex carbohydrates was from increased consumption of vegetables, fruit and wholegrain cereals. Over six menstrual cycles, there was a substantial reduction in pre-menstrual breast tenderness with the new diet. The improvement related not only to the reduction in fat and increase in fibre, but also to the increase in protein intake that occurred to make up the loss of fatty foods. Protein-rich foods tend to be high in vitamin B, iron, zinc and other nutrients. The effect of diet on other pre-menstrual symptoms was not, unfortunately, documented. The diet researched by the Women's Nutritional Advisory Service is similar, but not identical, to that used by Dr Boyd and his colleagues.

### Drug Treatments:

A useful and effective treatment for Pre-menstrual Tension, particularly with associated period pains, is mefenamic acid (Ponstan). Headaches, period pains and possibly breast pain, might be helped by such treatment, though mood swings and irritability may not always benefit. Two out of three studies have shown benefit with mefenamic acid, and these can be obtained on prescription.

**Diuretics:** A variety have been tried for PMT and pre-menstrual fluid retention. Most are not suitable for long-term usage, as they are either of limited effectiveness, cause increased losses of certain minerals, including magnesium, or when stopped may cause rebound fluid retention. One preparation of ammonium chloride and caffeine (Aquaban) has been shown to help prevent pre-menstrual weight gain, but such preparations may cause an aggravation of irritability and mental symptoms, and cannot be recommended as a general treatment. Probably the most effective treatment is with the diuretic, spironolactone (Aldactone) which can help fluid retention and other pre-menstrual symptoms, but again its use is not recommended in the long term. It might be considered as a short-term measure for those with particularly bad fluid retention symptoms, though a low-salt diet should always be used.

Vivienne was prescribed diuretics by her doctor because she was always so bloated.

*'They worked very well to start with, but as the years went on they had very little effect. I think my body must have got used to them.'*

**Psychiatric drugs** have also been used in PMT. The tranquillizer Lithium has not been shown to be effective. Certain sedatives, including meprobamate, alprazolam (Xanax), and buspirone (Buspar), have been shown to be effective, each in one study only. Only limited conclusions can therefore be drawn, in view of the potential problems with such drugs. Even the antibiotic, tetracycline, has been used, and shown to be effective in the treatment of PMT. It is more usually used in the treatment of acne, but it might be appropriate to consider its use if both conditions are a problem. Again, one should take care to pay attention to eating healthily.

Jane was prescribed Valium by her doctor.

> 'I tried Valium but it was no help, in fact it made me feel worse as it gave me panic attacks. I was on them for six months and then had difficulty stopping them. I went back to the doctor and just threw the tablets at him when I was pre-menstrual and said don't ever ever prescribe me that kind of tablet again as they made me feel so ill.'

Geraldine's life was pretty much at a standstill pre-menstrually. She couldn't function normally.

> 'My GP prescribed anti-depressants, which I took. I wasn't aware that they were helping me, but he kept telling me that they were. He kept telling me that they would help even though I wouldn't be aware of it! They did help me sleep a bit, but I was afraid I wouldn't wake up. They made me feel a bit zombie-like.'

### Hormonal Treatments:

Progesterone, the hormone that rises in the second half, luteal phase, of the menstrual cycle, has been subjected to at least four carefully conducted studies, none of which have achieved a positive outcome. The usual preparation, Cyclogest, has to be administered either as a pessary or suppository, or it can also be administered by injection. It is certainly no longer the first choice of hormonal treatment, despite its popularization by Dr Katharina Dalton. Progesterone in other forms may yet prove to be effective.

A synthetic progesterone, dydrogesterone (Duphaston), administered at a dosage of 10 mg twice daily in the last half of the menstrual cycle, was shown to be effective in two out of four studies. Mild to moderate benefit can be expected in some cases, with relatively few side-effects. Weight gain, however, can occur.

The oral contraceptive pill has a variable effect on PMT. Some women's symptoms may improve, others remain the same, and others worsen. It is very much hit and miss. Certainly for younger women who require oral contraception, or those who might require the oral contraceptive pill to help control heavy or irregular periods, this may be a useful approach. Again, it can be easily combined with dietary changes. The new lower dose, or phased dose, contraceptive pills seem to have substantially fewer side-effects than those used in the 1960s and 1970s. Serious side-effects, including an increased risk of stroke, may occur in cigarette smokers, the overweight, and those with high blood pressure, who are on the Pill.

Ruth was prescribed the contraceptive pill by her GP to help ease her problems.

*'After the birth of my first child, 14 years ago, my GP suggested I took the Pill for therapeutic reasons, to help remove the "tension" I was experiencing premenstrually. The Pill caused me awful headaches so I had to come off it. By this time my doctor had left the partnership and my new doctor prescribed vitamin B6. He wanted to try something natural before progesterone. I did not find that vitamin B6 made the slightest difference.'*

Implants of the hormone oestrogen have been used successfully in the control of PMT. This has the effect of retiring the ovaries, as the high level of oestrogen from the implant makes their activity redundant. This abolishes hormonal fluctuation, but is highly unnatural and expensive, and requires a small operation. This is best reserved for those with severely resistant PMT.

Other hormonal preparations including bromocriptine (Parlodel), danazol (Danol), and gonadotrophin-releasing hormone analogues have all been used successfully in the treatment of PMT. They usually are administered by doctors specializing in hormonal treatments. Again they are usually reserved for those with severe PMT that has failed to respond to other approaches.

As you can see from some of the case reports, different women will give different stories about different treatments. The most important factor is to find a treatment that suits you – your symptoms and your lifestyle.

If you are on any of the above drug or hormonal treatments, and they have not been successful for you, do not despair. Firstly, see your doctor about coming off, or changing your treatment. It may be easier to do this if you also make the dietary changes that we have been talking about, and make use of some of the nutritional supplements that are of proven effectiveness in the treatment of PMT.

Anita went back to her GP as the diuretics he had prescribed hadn't worked.

*'My doctor prescribed Primolut in massive doses. All it succeeded in doing was making me gain even more weight! There was a time five or six years ago when I tried Duphaston, but I didn't get on very well with that either. I felt I was given too much, and it seemed to exaggerate my symptoms.'*

As a last resort Ruth's GP prescribed Cyclogest pessaries for her to insert in her vagina.

*'I cannot remember how many I was told to take. They did work a little, but not enough. I got more and more tensed up nearer to my period. I was putting 12 pessaries up a day! They were awfully messy, and would come back down again anyway. If I had been more sane then I wouldn't have thought it was a good idea to stuff so many pessaries up. Finally, I was referred to a specialist who prescribed Duphaston, which did help. At least I could lead a normal life for a while, but PMT reared its ugly head again.'*

Pauline was given Duphaston by her GP.

*'After a few weeks I started to get breast tenderness. My breasts literally stood out and I was so uncomfortable. I began taking Aspro to help them feel more comfortable, but after two months the breast discomfort was even worse. I thought it was pointless to take one drug to ease the effects of another so I decided to stop taking them. I had dreadful problems coming off the Duphaston. I did come off gradually, but I have never known headaches like it and I had unbelievable sugar cravings.'*

## WOMEN'S NUTRITIONAL ADVISORY SERVICE STUDY – ON DRUG WITHDRAWAL IN 150 WOMEN

The number of women we came across who were taking tranquillizers or sleeping tablets was alarming, to say the least. Many of the women had been taking their drugs for years and admitted being addicted to them. It was interesting to note that, although they had been prescribed their drugs to overcome PMT and related problems, at the end of the day they still had to face the problem, but in a reduced state of awareness. And now they also had the side-effects of the drugs and the drug addiction to cope with.

Withdrawing from the drugs is a problem in itself: the withdrawal symptoms are often very disturbing and may need careful supervision. The demands on the body for extra nutrients during these withdrawals can be quite high. Thus we were initially surprised to see so many women coming off their drugs during the programme with no real difficulties. However, when we thought about the situation logically we understood the reasons for this. The fact is that all the women had been taking good amounts of vitamin and mineral supplements, while following a balanced diet through the duration of the programme. The extra level of nutrients probably helped the women over their symptoms, while also cushioning the usual withdrawal symptoms. Specific advice on drug withdrawals can be found on page 178.

On our study of 150 women, 93 of these were taking other medication at the time they began their programme, which consisted of tranquillizers, sleeping tablets and hormonal supplements. Seventy-five per cent of the women felt well enough to come off their drugs completely during the first three months of the programme. A further 16 per cent significantly reduced their medication and in fact only 9 per cent remained on their drugs.

I must emphasize that we did not suggest that any of the women stopped their medication. Our standard recommendation is for each patient to consult her doctor and to withdraw slowly from her drugs under medical supervision. Do not do it yourself but seek your doctor's advice and follow the dietary and supplement recommendations given later in the book, which may help you. Don't forget to tell your doctor about this too.

## DOCTOR'S APPROACH TO TREATMENT

Many experts now agree that the nutritional approach to treating the Pre-Menstrual Syndrome is the best first-line treatment. Whilst this is indeed a breakthrough, in theory the nutritional approach to PMT is not widely being applied.

In July 1989 the Women's Nutritional Advisory Service conducted a survey on 1000 UK doctors in order to become familiar with their prescribing habits, and their level of knowledge about nutrition.

Over half the doctors who responded to the survey (287) expressed difficulty when treating PMT.

Of the doctors in the survey, 70 per cent admitted having no nutritional training whatsoever, either as a medical student or as a postgraduate. A further 22 per cent admitted to minimal nutritional knowledge. It is indeed an ironic fact that 92 per cent of UK doctors feel that they are not equipped to administer what is considered by many experts to be the best first-line treatment for PMT.

The saving grace was that 79 per cent of the doctors in the survey said they would like to receive medical papers on the nutritional approach to PMT.

There is to this day inadequate training for doctors on nutrition in general, and the nutritional approach to PMT in particular, in the UK either for undergraduates or for doctors already qualified. Three-quarters of the women who contact the WNAS currently feel that their doctor does not really understand their problem, and does not offer helpful treatment.

We hope to be instrumental in reversing this situation in the 1990s.

# 13

# NUTRITION
# AND THE BODY:
# VITAMINS AND MINERALS,
# WHAT THEY DO

## THE BODY

One thing we have in common is that we all have a body! Our body is nothing more nor less than a highly complicated biochemical machine, the function of which, like any engine, is dependent upon the quality of its food or fuel supply. The body is composed of many different organs and tissues which have important and essential functions and interactions. For example, if you want to move your arm, a tiny electrical message passes from the brain, through the nervous system and down the nerves to the muscles in your arm, which then contract. The degree of stretch or tension in a muscle is relayed, via other nerves, back to the brain, so that the muscle does not over, or under stretch in performing the movement that you originally intended.

There are factors that affect the healthy function of nerves, muscles and all other parts of the body. *Firstly, you need to inherit a good and healthy metabolism*. The thousands of chemical processes that take place within each and every cell are mainly determined by the genetic material in the centre of the nucleus of the cell. This genetic material is a master plan or blueprint. It holds the key to which chemical reactions need to take place in order for that cell to function. It determines whether a cell is a muscle cell, nerve cell, skin cell, red blood cell, or any other type of cell. Almost everyone has healthy genes, and thus the possibility for their body to be completely healthy and function efficiently. However, there may be subtle individual variations in metabolism, which determine the strengths and weaknesses of one's physical constitution. This may explain why some people are sensitive to some types of dietary change or nutritional deficiencies, and others are not – why some women may develop Pre-Menstrual Tension, and others, despite eating an 'unhealthy' diet, may not.

*Secondly, some disease states can lead to the development of PMT.*

*Finally, and most importantly, there must be a healthy diet,* giving an adequate supply of those nutrients necessary for the normal functioning of each individual cell. A lack of any one nutrient leads to changes in the cell's metabolism, which in turn will result in changes in the individual's health.

## THE DIET

Many people, when they hear the word diet, think of a weight-reducing or slimming diet. The word diet simply refers to the type of food that a person is eating. Every one of us has a diet of some kind, unless we are starving to death. Certain components of a diet are essential, and many of these terms may be familiar to you. The essential nutrients include proteins, fats, carbohydrates, fibre, water, vitamins, minerals and essential fatty acids. Other factors that are also essential for life include a certain degree of heat and light. First, we should have a brief word about what each of these nutrients does, and why they are essential.

**Proteins.** These are the building blocks of a body. A protein is in fact a group of smaller building blocks called amino acids, which in turn are composed of individual chemicals. Proteins are found in large quantities in tissue such as muscle, skin and bone. In these tissues protein serves a mainly structural function, contributing to the shape of the body, and its ability to move. Other proteins perform highly specialized functions, such as hormones which influence metabolism, and antibodies which help to fight infection.

We all make our own proteins, mainly in the liver, but to do this, must have a steady supply, from our diet, of amino acids, which are in turn derived from the proteins that we eat. Thus, it is essential for us to eat good-quality proteins, such as fish, eggs, nuts, seeds, wholegrains, peas, beans and lentils and lean additive-free meat. A lack of protein in the diet would lead to loss of muscle function and performance, and to a multitude of changes in the body's metabolism.

**Fats.** These are providers of energy, and, apart from two essential fats (discussed below), are really not necessary to the body at all. However, every type of protein contains some fat, whether it is an animal or vegetable source of protein. This fat can be burnt by the body to provide energy. The liver and muscle cells in particular can make substantial use of fats in this way. Fats also provide a structural role in forming the walls of each individual cell.

The specialized fat, cholesterol, is used to form the male and female hormones, vitamin D and other important hormones in the body. Our bodies can usually make twice as much cholesterol as we eat. So often a raised level of cholesterol in the blood is caused not by eating too much cholesterol, but a faulty metabolism and a high-fat, high-sugar diet. We certainly do not need to increase our intake of animal fats, as I'm sure you will appreciate after reading the section on fats in Chapter 11, page 104.

**Essential fatty acids.** These are specialized fats, whose importance is becoming increasingly realized. There are two essential fatty acids, linoleic and linolenic acid. As their names suggest, they are very similar in chemical structure, and both of them are of the polyunsaturated type (i.e. not cholesterol-forming). These perform two main roles. First, they are a structural component of the walls of many cells, and thus contribute to the cellular skeleton of the body. Secondly, these two essential fatty acids can be transformed into a wide variety of different chemical compounds which appear to play a part in hormone function and inflammation. Disturbance in the metabolism of these essential fatty acids has been described in one group of women with PMT. However, this has not been confirmed by a second study. Even so, supplements of evening primrose oil, Efamol, have been shown to be effective in the treatment of PMT, as well as in the skin condition, eczema. It remains to be seen what role these nutrients play in PMT-causation.

**Carbohydrates.** Carbohydrates, too, are a source of energy. They can be divided into two categories: simple and complex. Simple ones include glucose, fructose (fruit sugar), sucrose (ordinary or table sugar), and lactose (milk sugar). Glucose and fructose are in fact the simplest sugars, consisting of only one type of sugar each. Sucrose and lactose, on the other hand, contain two different types of sugar joined together, and thus are sometimes known as di-saccharides (two-sugars).

Polysaccharides (literally, many sugars), are the 'complex' carbohydrates most usually found in vegetables. These consist of many interlinked sugar sub-units, and in order for them to be used by the body, they must be broken down into simple, single-sugar units by the digestive processes in the gut. Vegetables, wholegrains, nuts and seeds are high in these complex carbohydrates.

The refining of sugar cane and sugar beet to make table sugar, sucrose, results in a loss of some of these complex carbohydrates, and a loss in the vitamins, minerals and fibre present in the original plant. When we eat these carbohydrates they are converted by the digestive processes and the body's metabolism to the simple sugar, glucose, which is a major form of energy in the body. Glucose is essential for the brain, as it can only use this form of fuel. However, one does not have to eat glucose or sucrose, table sugar, in order for the brain and nervous system to have an adequate supply: the liver can make glucose from fats or proteins, as well as from other types of sugars, so while glucose is essential for life, it is a mistake to believe we have to add it to the diet. However, some form of carbohydrate, preferably the complex or unrefined carbohydrates, are necessary for an adequate supply of energy.

**Fibre.** Fibre is the undigestible carbohydrate residues found in food. Natural or unprocessed foods are usually high in fibre and include wholegrains, nuts, seeds and fruit. Some types of carbohydrate cannot be digested by the human body, and so pass through the stomach and digestive tract to the large bowel. Here, fibre absorbs water and other waste materials, and forms our waste product, faeces. A lack of fibre in the diet often leads to constipation, but it is now realized that fibre has other important functions. Lack of fibre is also associated with such conditions as gallstones, varicose veins, obesity, heart disease and diabetes. Of particular relevance is the fact that fibre binds with cholesterol and hormones that are secreted by the liver into the gut. A high-fibre diet may help in expulsion of excessive quantities of cholesterol and unwanted female sex hormones, but more of this later.

**Water.** This is of course essential for health. Our bodies are composed of 60–70 per cent water, and many bodily functions are dependent upon water. Water is necessary for vitamins, minerals and other chemicals to dissolve in. The amount of urine produced by the kidneys is largely dependent upon the amount of water consumed. An adequate water intake is necessary to clear waste materials through the kidneys, and to allow normal metabolic processes to take place. Water can sometimes be retained by the body, particularly if the intake of salt (sodium) is high. Both salt and water need to be cleared by the kidneys, and their ability to do this may vary from individual to individual. In our research, we have noticed that this may depend on a woman's nutritional state. Women who have suffered with pre-menstrual water retention for years, have managed to overcome the condition by making changes to their diet and taking additional supplements.

## VITAMINS

Vitamins are the best-known essential nutrient. Indeed, their name was derived from the term 'vital amines' (a type of chemical). They are named as letters of the alphabet, A, B, C, D, E, and K, and members of the B group are further subdivided by numbers into vitamins B1, 2, 3, 5, 6, 12 and Folic acid. The vitamins themselves, as a whole, are divided into two groups. The water-soluble vitamins include members of the vitamin B complex and vitamin C, and the fat-soluble group includes vitamins A, D, E and K.

123

Vitamins are vital but only in tiny or trace amounts, unlike proteins, carbohydrates and fats, which are necessary in substantial quantities. These trace amounts of vitamins help modify and control essential cellular reactions. Each vitamin which has particular relevance to the development of pre-menstrual symptoms is described in more detail below.

**Vitamin A.** This comes in two types: retinol (animal-derived), and beta-carotene (vegetable-derived). Deficiency of vitamin A is very rare indeed, and usually only occurs with a grossly inadequate diet or with severe impairment of digestive function. Supplements of vitamin A were used many years ago in the treatment of Pre-Menstrual Tension, apparently with good results, but very high doses were used, which could carry risk of serious side-effects. A lack of vitamin A usually results in an impairment of vision at night, or when in the dark. If deficiencies continue, there are further eye, as well as skin changes.

Recently, a number of studies have demonstrated that either poor intakes of vitamin A, or low blood levels, especially of beta-carotene, are associated with a future increased risk of certain types of cancer, including lung cancer. High intakes of fruit and vegetables rich in vitamin A may thus prove to have a cancer-protective effect.

**Vitamin B complex.** This is a group of several vitamins with certain things in common. They are all water-soluble, their metabolisms are often inter-related, and they are frequently found together in the same types of foods. Factors that lead to deficiency often, but not always, produce a deficiency of several of the vitamins in this group. Deficiency very often produces mental changes which have many similarities with those of Pre-Menstrual Tension.

**Vitamin B1, Thiamin,** is essential for the normal metabolism of sugar. Requirements for this vitamin increase if the diet is high in sugar, refined carbohydrates, and alcohol. Some substances which destroy thiamin are found in tea, coffee and raw fish. Good sources of this vitamin are wholegrains, most meats (preferably additive-free or organic) and beans. Any food that is refined is usually quite substantially depleted in thiamin. A lack of thiamin results in anxiety, depression, irritability, changes in behaviour, aggressiveness and loss of memory. These features may also be particularly marked in those consuming high quantities of alcohol. The recommended daily intake is 1–1.5 mg per day, higher levels being required by those women who lead more active lives and as a result consume more calories (kjs).

**Vitamin B2, Riboflavin,** is required for the metabolism of proteins, fats and carbohydrates, particularly in the liver. Deficiency rarely occurs as this vitamin is present in such a wide range of foods, including milk, cheese, meat, fish and some vegetables. Deficiency does not usually produce any mental symptoms. However, vitamin B2 is necessary for the metabolism of vitamin B6 (pyridoxine). Requirements are between 1.2 and 1.6 mg per day.

**Vitamin B3, Nicotinic Acid or Nicotinamide,** is essential for the metabolism of carbohydrates and the release of energy from them. It is found in brown rice, wheatgerm, peanuts and liver. Deficiency rarely occurs unless there is a very poor diet or a high intake of alcohol. In deficiency states, dry scaling and redness appear in light exposed areas, particularly the backs of hands, face, neck and top of the chest. Mental deterioration and diarrhoea are also features, but severe deficiency is very rare. Requirements are between 12 and 15 mg a day. B3 is present in yeast, liver, meat, poultry, legumes, wheat flour and corn. Eggs and milk contain a niacin equivalent called tryptophan.

**Vitamin B5, Pantothenic Acid,** has many important roles in metabolism. Deficiency rarely occurs, but symptoms of this include headaches, weakness, fatigue, emotional swings and muscle cramps. Poor diet or alcoholism is probably the cause of any deficiency. Pantothenic acid is found in a wide variety of wholesome foods, including most animal and vegetable sources of protein. Requirements are between 5 and 10 mg per day.

**Vitamin B6** comes in three different varieties: pyridoxine, pyridoxal and pyridoxamine. Pyridoxine is the sort normally used in vitamin supplements, and is also generally used in the treatment of Pre-Menstrual Tension. Vitamin B6 requires a supply of vitamin B2 – riboflavin – and magnesium before it is chemically active. Vitamin B6 plays a crucial role in the metabolism of proteins and in the normal metabolism of certain chemicals involved in the brain that control mood and behaviour. Good sources of vitamin B6 include most animal and vegetable proteins, especially fish, egg yolk, wholegrain cereals, nuts and seeds. Bananas, avocados, meat and some green leafy vegetables are also high in this nutrient. A McDonald's Big Mac hamburger contains only 0.02 mg of pyridoxine, which is only 1–2 per cent of that required per day. In fact, it does not contain enough vitamin B6 for the metabolism of the protein contained in the hamburger! Thus a diet containing a significant quantity of such depleted foods, will undoubtedly lead to vitamin B6 deficiency. Other factors which seem to affect it adversely include alcohol, the oral contraceptive pill and smoking. Deficiency of vitamin B6 produces anxiety, depression, loss of sense of responsibility and insomnia.

Some 15 per cent of women of childbearing age in the UK were recently found to have laboratory evidence of vitamin B6 deficiency. From the mid-1950s to the mid-1970s there was a 20 per cent reduction in vitamin B6 intakes, though in the

1980s this seemed to return to its higher level. There has also been increasing consumption of alcohol and increased usage of cigarettes and oral contraceptives amongst women of childbearing age over the last 30 years. All these factors tend to lower vitamin B6 levels and may contribute to some women's pre-menstrual symptoms.

**Vitamin B12 and Folic acid.** These two types of vitamin B are very important, particularly for the formation of blood and the functioning of nerves. Deficiencies tend to be rare. Vitamin B12 is found almost exclusively in animal produce, especially meat. Long-term vegetarians can be at risk of deficiency unless they take supplements.

Lack of Folic acid can occur from a poor diet, especially if you do not consume plenty of green, leafy vegetables. The name Folic acid comes from foliage, a major source of this important nutrient.

Increased requirements of vitamin B12 and Folic acid occur during pregnancy. Supplements of Folic acid are often given during pregnancy and vitamin B12 should be given to pregnant and breast-feeding mothers if they have been long-term strict vegetarians.

**Vitamin C.** Almost everyone knows that vitamin C deficiency causes scurvy, and we all think of scurvy as a disease of sailors in the past, and perhaps the extreme deprivation of Victorian times. Indeed, vitamin C deficiency is quite rare but still does occur in some elderly folk. However, in modern times, some people are at risk of having a lower level of vitamin C than is desirable for health. Smoking, in particular, reduces vitamin C levels substantially. The recommended daily intake in this country is only some 30 mg per day, about the amount in a apple. Considering cigarettes burn up this vitamin, 30 mg per day is a very low intake for a smoker. Some doctors feel that this intake should be higher: between 60 and 250 mg per day.

The increased intake of vitamin C may improve certain aspects of metabolism. In particular, the absorption of iron is helped by the presence of vitamin C in the food. Vitamin C is also necessary for the normal production of sex hormones and the breakdown of excess cholesterol in the body. The adrenal glands, two small glands just next to the kidneys, convert cholesterol into important hormones which control the metabolism of sugar, salt and water, as well as growth and tissue repair. The sex hormones oestrogen and progesterone originate mainly from the ovaries, but trace amounts also come from the adrenal glands. The adrenal glands have the highest concentration of vitamin C of any tissue in the body. The full importance of vitamin C has yet to be appreciated.

Deficiency of vitamin C produces depression, low energy and hypochondria, a condition in which the victim imagines he or she has a variety of different illnesses and complaints. Sometimes, an early sign of vitamin C deficiency is the presence of small pinpoint bruises under the tongue. This seems to be particularly common in smokers.

**Bioflavonoids.** Bioflavonoids (at one time known as vitamin P) are a group of different compounds found in high concentrations in citrus fruits, fruit, leafy vegetables, tea, coffee, wine, beer and to a lesser extent in root vegetables. It is mainly the skin, peel and outer layers of the fruit or vegetable which contains these compounds. Although they are not essential for health, they may have a variety of beneficial qualities including the strengthening of blood vessels, reducing inflammation and protecting against any damage caused by radiation. It does seem that a preparation containing vitamin C and bioflavonoids may help a woman with heavy periods. A supplement containing 600 mg of vitamin C, together with 600 mg of water-soluble bioflavonoid-compound produced a beneficial response in 14 out of 16 patients with excessive bleeding. Whether the benefit was due to the vitamin C or the bioflavonoids is uncertain, but other studies demonstrate that bioflavonoids may help strengthen the weakened blood vessels which may occur in people with varicose veins. This is yet another reason for eating plenty of fresh vegetables and fruit.

**Vitamin E.** Vitamin E is also known as tocopherol, from the Greek words meaning 'childbearing'. The name is given because rats deprived of vitamin E are unable to bear healthy offspring. Like vitamin C deficiency, vitamin E deficiency is also rare. There are no obvious symptoms or signs of its deficiency, but lack of it is likely to be caused by long-standing digestive problems. Supplements of vitamin E have also been used to treat Pre-Menstrual Syndrome and breast tenderness with some success. It is probable that extra vitamin E is not correcting a deficiency, but improving some aspect of metabolism. The normal daily requirements are in the region of 8–10 mg, which can usually be obtained from dietary sources such as vegetable oils, nuts, green vegetables, eggs and dairy produce.

Like vitamin A, recent evidence has appeared to suggest that low levels of vitamin E in women may be associated with an increased risk of breast cancer in later years. Again, ensuring a good intake of foods rich in such a vitamin may help you achieve good health, not only today, but also for your future tomorrows.

**Vitamin D.** Vitamin D is necessary for normal healthy bones and teeth. Most of us make adequate vitamin D if our skin is exposed to sunlight. Some can also be provided by the diet as in cod liver oil and dairy produce. Margarine in this country has vitamin D as well as vitamin A added to it. Vitamin D helps the body's absorption of calcium from the diet. In particular, it assists in the normal uptake of calcium into the bones and teeth to make them strong. Too much vitamin D can be toxic, more than 400 international units per day should not be consumed without medical advice.

## MINERALS

**Minerals** are essential components, and may be divided into two types. First there are those minerals which are required in substantial bulk quantities. These include calcium, phosphorus, magnesium, sodium and potassium. They play a large part in the formation of bones and cells. Some other minerals are required in only small amounts and are called trace elements. These include iron, zinc, copper, chromium, selenium and a variety of others. Their main function, like many vitamins, is to help stimulate the complex chemical reactions that take place in the body. A lack of these trace elements, rather like a lack of vitamins, can have a very wide-ranging dire effect upon the body's metabolism. Often the chemical reactions that control energy level and mood, as well as hormone function, can be adversely influenced.

**Calcium and Phosphorus.** These two minerals often go together, particularly in bones and teeth. It is important to have a good balance of calcium and phosphorus in the diet and the ratio of 2:1 is often recommended. Too much phosphorus will block the absorption of calcium and too much calcium will block the absorption of phosphorus. It is very rare that our diets lack phosphorus, but a lack of calcium is not so uncommon. Good sources of calcium include all dairy products, many nuts, especially Brazils and almonds, bony fish such as sardines, sprats and whitebait, beans, peas, lentils, wholegrains and some green vegetables, especially watercress. In fact, you do not have to eat dairy produce to get an adequate source of calcium but the rest of your diet must be very well balanced indeed. Recommended intakes vary between 500 mg and 1500 mg per day. The absorption of calcium is blocked by bran. Bran contains phytic acid, a substance that combines with calcium, preventing its absorption. (Indian chapattis may also have a similar effect.)

Many convenience foods contain phosphates in the form of food additives: soft drinks, including the low-calorie (kj) variety, are notoriously high in phosphate. As a high level interferes with calcium or magnesium balance, these products should be avoided as much as possible.

**Magnesium.** Magnesium seems to be a particularly important mineral as far as PMT is concerned. Firstly, magnesium, like calcium, is essential for healthy bones as well as nerves and muscles. Lack of magnesium produces poor appetite, nausea, apathy, weakness, tiredness, mood changes and muscle cramps. Good sources of magnesium include most wholefood, e.g. wholegrains, beans, peas, lentils, nuts, seeds and green vegetables. Water, particularly some bottled waters and tap water from a hard water area, can contain substantial quantities of this mineral, too.

In 1981 Dr Guy Abraham showed that a low level of magnesium was commonly found in women with PMT. Most of the magnesium is inside cells where it is busily involved in chemical reactions. Hence it is the level of magnesium inside the cells – red blood cell magnesium – and not the magnesium in the water compartment of blood that is often low. We repeated his work on magnesium deficiency in 105 women with PMT and showed that some 45 per cent of women had evidence of magnesium deficiency. We don't know precisely how important this deficiency is, but it seems likely that it has an effect on our mental function, the control of the levels of blood sugar and energy, and also the metabolism of some hormones. Unfortunately, there may be no obvious physical signs of magnesium deficiency and so it is easily missed.

Interestingly in the UK, the intake of magnesium from food provided in the home only just achieves that recommended by most authorities. Intake should be in the region of 250–400 mg per day, and only reaches 249 mg per day per person in the average British household's food supply. Like calcium, requirements increase substantially during pregnancy and while breast-feeding, and it is often after a pregnancy and breast-feeding that the worst cases of magnesium deficiency are seen. This may well explain why some women's pre-menstrual problems begin shortly after childbirth. Indeed, magnesium deficiency is also associated with some other problems such as poor contractions of the womb during labour, elevated blood pressure during pregnancy and pre-eclamptic toxaemia. These conditions can be treated by injections of magnesium, an approach often used in the US, but not so much in the UK.

It is important that women with PMT consume a diet rich in magnesium. Sometimes your doctor can arrange for a simple red cell magnesium test to be performed at the local hospital and this may serve as a guide to the use of magnesium supplements.

**Sodium and Potassium.** These two minerals form an interesting pair. Both sodium and potassium are essential for the normal functioning of almost all cells in the body, particularly nerves and muscles. Since the use of more convenience foods, our diets have had markedly increased levels of sodium. Although table salt and sea salt (both are sodium chloride) represent a substantial source of sodium in our diets, most of the sodium we consume is found in convenience and other tinned, frozen or prepared foods.

Potassium is found mainly in fruit and vegetables, particularly tomatoes, bananas, figs, citrus fruits and almost all green leafy vegetables. Most of the potassium is found inside the cells rather like magnesium, and most of the sodium is found outside the cells. It is the balance of sodium and potassium that is important. This balance has to be maintained: if it is not, then the body may retain water. Too much sodium in the diet is indeed the commonest cause of fluid retention in many women, particularly in the week or so before the start of a period.

129

Water tablets, known as diuretics, will get rid of this excess fluid retention, but after a while the system gets used to them and the fluid retention returns, sometimes even worse than before. As well as getting rid of the excess water in the body, diuretics have the effect of ridding the body of useful potassium and magnesium, which makes the situation worse.

The answer: reduce sodium intake in the diet by not having salt at the table, not using it in the cooking, and avoiding any salty foods. It is difficult, on the contrary, to consume too much potassium, and problems only arise in patients with kidney disease.

**Iron.** Iron is one of the most important trace minerals. We all know that iron is necessary for healthy blood and a lack of it results in anaemia. Iron is necessary for the formation of the blood pigment haemoglobin. What is not widely appreciated is that iron is also found in high concentrations in muscles and in the brain. It is necessary for the uptake of energy by muscles as well as for certain aspects of mental function in the normal brain. Iron deficiency is probably the most common deficiency in the world. Women, of course, have increased needs for iron because of their monthly blood-loss due to menstruation. Women who have heavy periods, such as those using the coil, may automatically have increased requirements.

Good sources of iron include wholefoods such as peas, beans, lentils, nuts, seeds and wholegrains, eggs, meat and to a lesser extent fish. The iron from animal sources is easily absorbed, whereas iron from vegetarian sources may not be so well absorbed, particularly if tea and coffee are consumed at the same meal. Vitamin C in the diet may greatly assist the absorption of iron from vegetarian foods.

The features of iron deficiency include fatigue, tiredness, digestive problems, poor quality nails, and recurrent infections, especially thrush. Although 10 per cent of women of childbearing age are at risk of developing these problems due to iron deficiency, only one-fifth of these women will actually be anaemic. This means that to detect iron deficiency the doctor must not just measure the haemoglobin level but actually measure the level of iron in the blood for a protein associated with iron called ferritin. If you think you are iron deficient *don't* rely upon your own doctor just doing a test to see if you are anaemic. The iron level or ferritin level must be measured and any deficiency treated. Of course, the most sensible thing to do is to eat a well-balanced diet and avoid the factors that can lead to iron-deficiency. It is a good idea not to drink tea and coffee immediately after meals, but only drink it two hours before or after eating.

Any women with continually heavy periods should have this problem looked into. In fact iron deficiency can even be a cause of heavy periods. Now you can see how important a trace mineral can be!

**Zinc.** Zinc, like iron, affects many different aspects of metabolism, particularly those involved in growth, and resistance to infection. It is necessary for healthy skin, normal hormone production and normal mental function. Adequate quantities can be obtained from wholegrains, nuts, peas, beans, lentils and meat. Like iron, zinc absorption may be blocked by tea and coffee as the tannin from the drink binds with it, preventing its absorption. You know what strong tea can do to the inside of a white teacup – imagine what it does to the inside of your intestines!

Anyone regularly consuming substantial quantities of alcohol, i.e. more than two glasses of wine or a pint of beer per day, is at risk of developing zinc as well as vitamin B deficiencies. Women on the Pill can have lower levels of zinc, as can those who make long-term use of diuretics – water pills. Often a useful clue to a lack of zinc is poor quality skin such as excessively dry or greasy facial skin, particularly at the sides of the nose. Eczema, acne and psoriasis may also suggest a deficiency of this important mineral. Another physical sign can be white spots on the nails, though this is not always reliable. Interestingly, the metabolism of zinc and vitamin B6 are closely related, which explains why the skin changes produced by these two deficiencies can have a similar appearance.

**Copper.** Copper is needed for energy metabolism, particularly by the liver. Deficiency is rare and is certainly unlikely to be encountered in women, as the female sex hormone oestrogen tends to increase copper levels in the blood. Indeed, oral contraception-users have higher copper and lower zinc levels than those who do not use the Pill. There is usually no need to take copper supplements and any multi-vitamin/multi-mineral preparation containing copper should have an adequate quantity of zinc with it. One side-effect, however, of taking large quantities of zinc – more than 30 mg per day for several months – is that it can lead to copper deficiency, but this is very rare.

**Chromium.** Chromium is a fascinating trace mineral. Only minute quantities are required: a lifetime's supply of chromium only weighs one-sixth of an ounce (5 g), and the body will only use 1 per cent of that. Yet even this tiny amount of chromium plays a crucial part in the control of blood sugar metabolism. A lack of chromium can lead to poor blood-sugar control, which in turn can lead to fluctuating energy levels and the dreaded sugar cravings. They are a classic feature of some women's pre-menstrual symptoms, as we have seen.

In severe cases of chromium deficiency a diabetes-like state can occur, particularly in older people. Chromium supplements can have a marked effect in this situation, and can also help improve poor blood-sugar control in people who are not diabetics. Eating large quantities of carbohydrates such as table sugar increases the loss of chromium in the urine. There are no outward signs of chromium

131

deficiency, unless you count the presence of old sweet wrappers in the bottom of your handbag! We have seen no end of 'little miracles' as a result of increasing chromium intake: it really is very useful in helping to control the sugar cravings. Eating a sensible diet is the best way to prevent chromium deficiency. Foods which contains a good quantity of chromium are green vegetables, root vegetables, eggs, scallops, shrimps, rye and some fruit.

That ends all you really need to know about vitamins and minerals. It may be useful to summarize this vital information and indicate how you can recognize any deficiencies.

## VITAMINS AND MINERALS – DO YOU LACK THEM?

| | Food Sources | What They Do |
|---|---|---|
| Vitamin B6 | *Meat, fish, nuts, bananas, avocados, wholegrains.* | *Essential in the metabolism of protein and the amino acids that control mood and behaviour. Affects hormone metabolism.* |
| Vitamin B1 Thiamin | *Meat, fish, nuts, wholegrains.* | *Essential in the metabolism of sugar, especially in nerves and muscles.* |
| Vitamin C Ascorbic acid | *Any fresh fruits and vegetables.* | *Involved in healing, repair of tissues and production of some hormones.* |
| Iron | *Meat, wholegrains, nuts, eggs.* | *Essential to make blood – haemoglobin. Many other tissues need iron for energy reactions.* |
| Zinc | *Meat, wholegrains, nuts, peas, beans, lentils.* | *Essential for normal growth, mental function, hormone production and resistance to infection.* |
| Magnesium | *Green vegetables, wholegrains, Brazil and almond nuts, many other non-junk foods.* | *Essential for sugar and energy metabolism, needed for healthy nerves and muscles.* |

132

As a general rule vitamin and mineral deficiencies are caused by a poor diet or the presence in the diet of agents such as alcohol, tea, coffee, cigarettes, poor-quality food, or an excessive consumption of carbohydrates. These increase the need for nutrients from the remaining healthy foods that are consumed. If you have any symptoms or signs of deficiencies which persist despite a healthy diet, or despite taking nutritional supplements for a period of three months, then it is important to consult your medical practitioner. In the Self-Help section on diet, beginning on page 137, more attention will be given to the foods which are high in essential vitamins and minerals and how to have a diet with sufficient quantities of each.

## Deficiencies

| Who is at Risk | Symptoms | Visible Signs |
|---|---|---|
| Women, especially those on the Pill, breast-feeding mothers, smokers, 'junk-eaters'. | Depression Anxiety Insomnia Loss of responsibility. | Dry/greasy facial skin, cracking at corners of the mouth. |
| Alcohol consumers, women on the Pill, breast-feeding mothers, high consumers of sugar. | Depression Anxiety, Poor appetite, Nausea Personality change. | None usually! Heart, nerve and muscle problems if severe. |
| Smokers particularly. | Lethargy Depression Hypochondriasis (imagined illnesses). | Easy bruising, look for small pin-point bruises under the tongue. |
| Women who have heavy periods (e.g. coil users), vegetarians, especially if tea or coffee drinkers, women with recurrent thrush. | Fatigue, poor energy, depression, poor digestion, sore tongue, cracking at corners of mouth. | Pale complexion, brittle nails, cracking at corners of mouth. |
| Vegetarians, especially tea and coffee drinkers, alcohol consumers, long-term users of diuretics – water pills. | Poor mental function, skin problems in general, repeated infections. | Eczema, acne, greasy or dry facial skin, white spots on nails. |
| Women with PMT! (some 50 per cent may be lacking), long-term diuretic users, alcohol consumers. | Nausea, apathy, loss of appetite, depression, mood changes, muscle cramps. | Usually NONE! so easily missed; muscle spasms sometimes. |

## TRIED AND TESTED

The value of the nutritional approach to PMT can be measured in a laboratory. Here are three examples of patients who had 'before' and 'after' laboratory tests. These tests allow us to measure vitamin and mineral levels to verify precise deficiencies which can then be treated.

## GERALDINE ELLIS

Geraldine had mainly been troubled by PMT D, and episodes of recurrent thrush. In the past, taking the oral contraceptive pill had aggravated her thrush and worsened her feelings of depression, but stopping the Pill had not stopped the thrush. Similarly, nutritional deficiencies can pre-dispose to thrush, especially a deficiency of iron, and Geraldine was quite severely iron-deficient. The level of iron in her blood was 2 micromols per litre, normal range being 11–29. She was iron-deficient even though she was not anaemic. Iron is necessary, not just for making the blood pigment haemoglobin, but also because it helps to strengthen muscles and improves the digestive system and the ability of cells to fight infection.

Treatment with supplements of iron, multi-vitamins and a further course of anti-fungal treatment to control her thrush resulted in a substantial improvement in Geraldine's pre-menstrual symptoms, clearance of her thrush and correction of the iron deficiency itself. She also had a low level of magnesium in the red cells so required an additional magnesium supplement.

## SANDRA PATTERSON

Sandra was a 29-year-old, single girl for whom Pre-Menstrual Tension carried a very special significance: on two occasions pre-menstrually she had inadvertently shoplifted. In her pre-menstrual confusion she had forgotten to pay for goods as she left the shop. The mistake was picked up by the store detective before she herself had time to return to the shop and pay for them. The courts put her on probation the first time and Sandra decided she must do something about the Pre-Menstrual Tension. She started taking Efamol evening primrose oil, 500 mg capsules, four per day. This controlled her pre-menstrual symptoms extremely well, so well in fact that after a few months she stopped them altogether. Unfortunately, the next month her PMT returned and with it her second shoplifting episode. The court was now beginning to find her story hard to believe.

134

In fact, the laboratory investigations showed that Sandra had some marked nutritional deficiencies of zinc and vitamin B6. The activity of vitamin B6 in her blood was 46 per cent below an optimum level, the normal range being up to 15 per cent below – this indicated a severe deficiency. Similarly, the level of zinc was also depressed by some 25 per cent. Both zinc and vitamin B6 deficiencies may have influenced mental function and mood. Both play a crucial part in the metabolism of essential fatty acids, a specialized form of which is found in evening primrose oil. Thus it was that evening primrose oil was controlling Sandra's symptoms, without correcting all the underlying nutritional deficiencies. When an appropriate supplement of zinc and vitamin B6 was combined with her evening primrose oil, her pre-menstrual symptoms once again disappeared completely. With a better diet she was able to reduce her need for nutritional supplements. Fortunately the court took a lenient attitude on the second occasion, and she is now well aware of the responsibility she has to look after herself.


## REBECCA HARLEY

Rebecca had a long history of Pre-Menstrual Tension and low energy levels which showed a significant improvement when her nutritional problems were treated. Investigations showed her to have a very low level of magnesium. The red cell value was 1.5 millimols per litre, normal range being 2–3. Treatment with magnesium supplements, multi-vitamins (especially vitamin B6) and avoiding salt and wheat, made a substantial reduction in her symptoms of PMT H, fluid retention, abdominal bloating, as well as her other symptoms of anxiety, depression and fatigue. However, the fatigue was persistent and she had a rather puffy facial appearance. This suggested that the thyroid gland might be under-active. First tests were normal, but repeat tests a few months later showed that the thyroid was indeed beginning to fail. The pituitary gland, at the base of the brain, normally produces a thyroid stimulation hormone known as TSH. The TSH level had increased to 5.2 micro units per litre, when the normal value should be less than 5. Thus the pituitary gland was producing slightly increased amounts of hormone to try to stimulate the failing thyroid. Treatment with small quantities of thyroid hormone made a dramatic difference to Rebecca's symptoms. Finally, her magnesium level rose to 2.55 millimols per litre, thus showing full correction of the deficiency. An underactive thyroid should always be considered in women with Pre-Menstrual Tension, especially PMT H symptoms which do not respond to other treatment. An underactive thyroid may be the underlying cause not only of PMT, but also of heavy periods, a lack of periods, weight gain, decreased energy level, depression, mental sluggishness and dry skin.

## RESULTS OF THE NUTRITIONAL PROGRAMME

Although we were encouraged by the results we were achieving using the Nutritional Programme, we felt that we should measure the success more scientifically. In July 1985 we looked at a group of 150 PMT sufferers who had followed the recommendations we made. We also looked at a group of 25 women who had partially followed the programme. Some of the results are given below.

| 150 women who followed the recommendations | 25 women who partially followed the recommendations |
| --- | --- |
| 91 per cent reduction of severe symptoms over a three-month period. | 85 per cent reduction of severe symptoms over a three-month period. |
| 87 per cent of women reported that they were significantly better after three months. | 72 per cent of women reported that they were significantly better after three months. |

In November 1988 we repeated this analysis on 200 patients who were on our nutritional programme, and taking the supplement Optivite. Of the women analysed, 96.5 per cent considered that they had no symptoms or that their symptoms were almost completely gone or significantly improved after three months.

From the analysis of the results of the programme, we drew the following conclusions:

1) The individual dietary, supplement and exercise programme seemed highly effective for severe to moderate PMT sufferers.

2) There was a correlation between the degree to which the patient followed the recommendations and her results. In other words, if she followed the programme closely, she should achieve better results than someone only partially following the programme.

3) The programme seemed effective for women who had previously tried other methods of treatment for their PMT.

In Part Three, I will be looking closely at those factors in the diet which seem to be causing problems, and explain why.

The mere fact that so many women seem to make a miraculous recovery from their PMT in such a short space of time certainly indicates that all is not well with our diet, and that as a nation we are sadly lacking in sound dietary education.

# 14

# CHOOSING A
# NUTRITIONAL PLAN

The Nutritional Approach to PMT is one which involves making dietary and lifestyle changes. It may span a very broad spectrum, in that mild sufferers may only need to make a few dietary changes, whilst the moderate and severe sufferers need to follow a more specialized diet and perhaps even change their lifestyle to some degree.

In order to accommodate all PMT sufferers, I have prepared three options for you to choose from:

**Option 1**   Basic dietary and health recommendations – for mild sufferers.

**Option 2**   A specialized dietary plan – for moderate sufferers.

**Option 3**   A tailor-made nutritional programme – for moderate and severe sufferers.

Be guided by the severity of symptoms when making your choice of option, and not the convenience of one regime as opposed to another!

The closer you stick to the recommendations, the better your chances of rapid improvement. It's worth bearing this in mind as you go along, especially if you find it hard going making some of the changes.

### OPTION 1 – BASIC DIETARY AND
### HEALTH RECOMMENDATIONS

1.  **Reduce intake of sugar and 'junk' foods.** This includes sugar added to tea and coffee, sweets, cakes, chocolates, biscuits, puddings, jams, marmalade, soft drinks, ice cream and honey. Consumption of these

foods may cause water retention and block the uptake of essential minerals.

2.  **Reduce intake of salt, both added during the cooking and at the table.** Also reduce the intake of salty foods, e.g. salted nuts, kippers, bacon, etc. This causes fluid retention and may contribute to other PMT symptoms.

3.  **Reduce intake of tea and coffee.** Consume no more than one or two cups of tea and coffee per day. There are many pleasant herbal teas and substitutes for coffee from healthfood shops.

4.  **Eat green vegetables or salad daily.** A good helping of either of these should be obtained and eaten every day. Both of these contain important vitamins and minerals useful in the treatment of PMT symptoms.

5.  **Limit your intake of dairy products.** They interfere with magnesium absorption, a mineral which is often deficient in PMT sufferers. Restrict yourself to only one serving a day to be safe.

6.  **Reduce intake of tobacco and alcohol.** These aggravate some PMT symptoms.

7.  **Use good vegetable oils.** A good-quality vegetable oil, such as sunflower or safflower seed oil, should be used for any cooking, or for making salad dressings. Similarly, a sunflower seed margarine should be used rather than butter or other margarine.

8.  **Eat plenty of wholefoods.** By 'wholefoods' we mean foods, usually of vegetable origin, which have not been processed or refined, e.g. wholemeal bread and cereals, such as rye, oats, barley and millet. Food such as nuts and seeds are high in vitamins and minerals as too are the important vegetable oils. If eating meat, make sure that it is lean, and eat fish and poultry too. Certain fish, e.g. herring and salmon, contain some essential oils which are helpful in maintaining skin quality and may be of some value in preventing pre-menstrual breast tenderness.

9.  **Have regular exercise.** Physical exercise is of proven value in the treatment of pre-menstrual symptoms. Certainly those with a sedentary job, particularly those who do not get into the fresh air, should take regular physical exercise. Exercise, fresh air and exposure to sunlight are important factors in maintaining health, just as important as ensuring a healthy diet and taking vitamin and mineral supplements.

10. **Take a walk.** In moments of pure desperation or impending aggression, please do immediately take a walk. Get out of the house and change your

environment. Walk quietly, taking notice of the things around you. Do this until you feel a bit better.

## OPTION 2 – A SPECIALIZED DIETARY PLAN

As well as following the broad dietary recommendations outlined in Option 1 you will need to select a diet that will help your particular symptoms. Once you have worked out which vitamins and minerals you need to concentrate on from the chart below, you can then go on to refer to the food lists and menus that apply to you.

## BROAD DIETARY REQUIREMENTS
## FOR PMT AND OTHER RELATED SYMPTOMS

**PMT A** – **nervous tension, mood swings, irritability and anxiety.** Sufferers need high vitamin B6 and magnesium diets.

**PMT H** – **weight gain, swelling of extremities, breast tenderness and abdominal bloating.** Sufferers need high vitamin E, vitamin B6 and magnesium diets.

**PMT C** – **headache, craving for sweets, increased appetite, heart pounding, fatigue and dizziness or fainting.** Sufferers need high vitamin B6, magnesium and chromium diets.

**PMT D** – **depression, forgetfulness, crying, confusion and insomnia.** Sufferers need high vitamin B6, magnesium and vitamin C diets.

**Acne/skin problems.** A diet high in zinc is needed.

**Smokers.** Need high vitamin C diets.

**Anaemic/heavy periods.** Need high iron diets.

If, for example, you decide you are suffering with PMT A (Anxiety) and PMT C (Sugar Cravings) you will need to concentrate on a diet high in vitamin B6, magnesium and chromium. You simply refer to the relevant food lists on the following pages when selecting the foods to include in your daily diet. The sample menu plan for one week follows the food lists. This is designed to give you a guide to balanced menu planning. It's not something you have to follow, but you might like to use it as a starting point.

## WHERE TO SHOP

I will be suggesting that you eat plenty of salads, vegetables and fruit. You will have realized from Chapter 11 in Part Two that many of these foods are contaminated with chemicals. Fortunately, most of the large supermarkets are now beginning to stock organic produce. Although this is a little more expensive, if you can possibly manage to buy it, you'll be better off. That is, unless you grow your own organic produce, which makes even more sense.

Whilst there are many vegetarian suggestions and recipes included, I have catered for meat and fish eaters as well. Again, because of the chemicals and drugs in meat, I would suggest you try to find a butcher who will buy additive-free meat for you from an organic farm.

Changing over to a full range of organic produce is going to take some time. Currently the demands by retailers for organic produce cannot be met. As more and more farmers switch, there will be plenty to go round.

## A SAMPLE MENU PLAN FOR ONE WEEK

B = Breakfast   L = Lunch   D = Dinner   S = Sweet
Recipes in Chapter 16, p 179.

### DAY 1

B   Orange juice
    Muesli (home-made) with
        milk

L   Broccoli soup
    1 slice of wholemeal
        (wholewheat) bread

D   Mackerel with herbs (foil-baked)
    Brown rice salad
    Apple and celery salad

S   Baked pears with raisins

### DAY 2

B   Fresh grapefruit and orange salad
        with sunflower seeds
    Toast and dried fruit conserve or
        sugar-free jam (jelly)

L   Stuffed peppers (bell peppers)
    Banana

D   Roast chicken
    Cabbage
    Turnips
    Swede (rutabaga) and carrot mix
    Sliced fried potatoes

S   Slice of date and walnut cake

## DAY 3

B   Apple juice
Poached egg and toast

L   Lentil and vegetable soup
Avocado with crab meat or
   prawns (shrimps)
Green bean salad
Fresh orange

D   Lamb paprika
Brown rice

S   Stuffed baked apple

## DAY 4

B   Wholewheat pancakes (crêpes)
$\frac{1}{2}$ quantity dried fruit conserve
$\frac{1}{2}$ grapefruit

L   Jacket potatoes with tuna
Bulgar (cracked wheat) and nut
   salad
Orange and cucumber salad
Slice of melon

D   Steamed fish with garlic, spring
   (green) onions and ginger
Stir-fried vegetables

S   Rhubarb fool

## DAY 5

B   Orange juice
Scrambled eggs and tomatoes
   with toast

L   Grilled sardines
1 slice wholemeal (wholewheat)
   bread
Beanshoot salad
Grapes

D   Nut roast
Brown rice
Waldorf salad

S   Fresh fruit salad

## DAY 6

B   Grapefruit juice
Yogurt with sliced apple and
   raisins

L   Nutty parsnip soup
Cheese omelette
Red cabbage, apple and bean
   salad
Plums

D   Liver with orange
Leafy green vegetables
Boiled potatoes
Cauliflower and carrots

S   Ginger bananas

## DAY 7

B   Apple juice
Poached haddock
Tomatoes and mushrooms

L   Cauliflower and leeks in cheese
   sauce
Slice of bread
Orange

D   Vegetarian goulash
Brown rice

S   Fresh fruit salad

141

# NUTRITIONAL CONTENT OF FOOD PER 100g (4oz)

*Foods containing vitamin B6*

|  | mg |
| --- | --- |
| **Cereals** | |
| Wholemeal (wholewheat) flour | 0.50 |
| Wheat bran | 1.38 |
| Soya flour low fat | 0.68 |

| **Meat** | |
| --- | --- |
| Bacon (lean) | 0.45 |
| Gammon (lean) | 0.37 |
| Beef forerib (lean only) | 0.33 |
| Minced (ground) beef (stewed) | 0.30 |
| Lamb breast (roast lean only) | 0.22 |
| Veal (roast) | 0.32 |
| Chicken (roast meat only) | 0.26 |
| Duck (roast meat only) | 0.25 |
| Turkey (roast meat only) | 0.32 |
| Liver (stewed) | 0.64 |

| **Fish** | |
| --- | --- |
| Cod (baked) | 0.38 |
| Cod (grilled) | 0.41 |
| Salmon (steamed) | 0.83 |
| Plaice (steamed) | 0.47 |
| Herring (grilled) | 0.57 |
| Kipper (baked) | 0.57 |
| Mackerel (fried) | 0.84 |

| **Fruit** | |
| --- | --- |
| Bananas (raw) | 0.51 |
| Apricots dried (raw) | 0.17 |
| Prunes dried (raw) | 0.24 |
| Raisins dried | 0.30 |

|  | mg |
| --- | --- |
| **Vegetables and pulses** | |
| Butter (lima) beans (raw) | 0.58 |
| Haricot beans (raw) | 0.56 |
| Mung beans (raw) | 0.50 |
| Red kidney beans (raw) | 0.44 |
| Broccoli tops (boiled) | 0.13 |
| Brussels sprouts (boiled) | 0.17 |
| Cabbage red (raw) | 0.21 |
| Cauliflower (boiled) | 0.12 |
| Avocado pear | 0.42 |
| Leeks (boiled) | 0.15 |
| Potatoes (boiled and baked) | 0.18 |

| **Nuts** | |
| --- | --- |
| Hazelnuts | 0.55 |
| Peanuts | 0.50 |
| Walnuts | 0.73 |

| **Other** | |
| --- | --- |
| Tomato purée (paste) | 0.63 |
| Bovril (Miso) | 0.53 |
| Marmite (Miso) | 1.3 |

*Foods containing magnesium*

| **Cereals** | |
| --- | --- |
| Wheat bran | 520 |
| Wholemeal (wholewheat) flour | 140 |
| Oatmeal (raw) | 110 |
| Porridge (rolled) oats | 30 |
| Soya flour (low fat) | 290 |
| Wholemeal (wholewheat) bread | 230 |
| Muesli | 100 |

142

## Dairy

| | mg |
|---|---|
| Dried skimmed (skim) milk | 117 |
| Fresh whole milk | 12 |

## Meat

| | |
|---|---|
| Beef (lean cooked) | 11 |
| Lamb (lean cooked) | 12 |
| Chicken meat (roast) | 24 |
| Sheep's heart (roast) | 35 |

## Fish

| | |
|---|---|
| Cod (baked) | 26 |
| Herring (grilled) | 32 |
| Kipper (baked) | 48 |
| Pilchards (canned) | 39 |
| Salmon (steamed) | 29 |
| Sardines (canned in oil) | 52 |
| Winkles (boiled) | 360 |
| Crab (boiled) | 48 |

## Fruit (raw)

| | |
|---|---|
| Pineapple (fresh) | 17 |
| Apricots (fresh) | 12 |
| Apricots (dried) | 65 |
| Bananas | 42 |
| Blackberries | 30 |
| Dates (dried) | 59 |
| Figs (dried) | 92 |
| Raisins (dried) | 42 |
| Passion-fruit | 39 |
| Sultanas (golden raisins) | 35 |
| Prunes (dried) | 27 |

## Nuts

| | |
|---|---|
| Almonds | 260 |
| Brazil | 410 |
| Walnuts | 130 |
| Peanuts | 180 |

## Vegetables and Pulses

| | mg |
|---|---|
| Butter (lima) beans (boiled) | 33 |
| Haricot beans (boiled) | 45 |
| Mung beans (raw) | 170 |
| Chick peas (dahl) (cooked) | 67 |
| Spinach (boiled) | 59 |
| Sweetcorn (boiled) | 45 |
| Potatoes baked (with skins) | 24 |
| Avocado pear | 29 |

## Beverages/drinks

| | |
|---|---|
| Infusion sachet | 6 |
| Indian tea | 250 |

## Other

| | |
|---|---|
| Black treacle (molasses) | 140 |

*Foods containing zinc*

## Cereals

| | |
|---|---|
| Wheat bran | 16.2 |
| Wholemeal (wholewheat) flour | 3.0 |

## Dairy

| | |
|---|---|
| Milk whole | 0.35 |
| Dried whole milk | 3.2 |
| Dried skimmed (skim) milk | 4.1 |
| Cheddar cheese | 4.0 |
| Parmesan cheese | 4.0 |
| Yogurt | 0.60 |

## Eggs

| | |
|---|---|
| Eggs (boiled) | 1.5 |
| Egg yolk (raw) | 3.6 |
| Egg (poached) | 1.5 |

mg

## Meat

| | |
|---|---|
| Bacon (cooked) | 0.8 |
| Beef (lean roast) | 6.8 |
| Lamb (cooked) | 1.4 |
| Lamb chops (lean only grilled) | 4.1 |
| Pork (grilled lean only) | 3.5 |
| Chicken (roast meat) | 1.4 |
| Turkey (roast meat) | 2.4 |
| Liver (fried) | 6.0 |

## Nuts

| | |
|---|---|
| Almonds | 3.1 |
| Brazils | 4.2 |
| Hazelnuts | 2.4 |
| Peanuts | 3.0 |
| Walnuts | 3.0 |

## Fish

| | |
|---|---|
| Cod (baked) | 0.5 |
| Plaice (fried) | 0.7 |
| Herring (grilled) | 0.5 |
| Mackerel (fried) | 0.5 |
| Salmon (canned) | 0.9 |
| Sardines (canned in oil) | 3.0 |
| Tuna (canned) | 0.8 |
| Crab (boiled) | 5.5 |
| Prawns (shrimps) (boiled) | 2.1 |
| Oysters (raw) | 45.0 |
| Mussels (boiled) | 2.1 |

## Vegetables and Pulses

| | |
|---|---|
| Butter (lima) beans (boiled) | 1.0 |
| Savoy cabbage (boiled) | 0.2 |
| Cabbage red (raw) | 0.3 |
| Lentils split (boiled) | 1.0 |
| Peas fresh (boiled) | 0.5 |
| Lettuce | 0.2 |
| Spinach (boiled) | 0.4 |
| Sweetcorn (boiled) | 1.0 |

mg

## Other

| | |
|---|---|
| Ginger (ground) | 6.8 |

*Foods containing iron*

## Cereals

| | |
|---|---|
| Bemax (wheat germ) | 10.0 |
| Wheat bran | 12.9 |
| Rice | 0.5 |

## Meat

| | |
|---|---|
| Beef (lean cooked) | 1.4 |
| Rumpsteak (boneless sirloin) (lean only grilled) | 3.5 |
| Lamb (lean roast) | 2.5 |
| Lamb kidney | 12.0 |
| Pork lean (grilled) | 1.2 |
| Pig liver (stewed) | 17.0 |
| Veal | 1.2 |
| Chicken (dark meat) | 1.0 |
| Chicken (liver fried) | 9.1 |
| Bovril (Miso) | 14.0 |

## Eggs

| | |
|---|---|
| Eggs whole (boiled) | 2.0 |
| Egg yolk (raw) | 6.1 |

## Fish

| | |
|---|---|
| Mackerel (fried) | 1.2 |
| Sardines (canned in oil) | 2.9 |
| Trout (steamed) | 1.0 |
| Crab (boiled) | 1.3 |
| Prawns (shrimps) (boiled) | 1.1 |
| Cockles (boiled) | 26.0 |
| Mussels (boiled) | 7.7 |
| Oysters (raw) | 6.0 |
| Scallops (steamed) | 3.0 |

|  | mg |
|---|---|
| **Nuts** | |
| Almonds | 4.2 |
| Brazils | 2.8 |
| Coconut (fresh) | 2.1 |

| | mg |
|---|---|
| **Dairy** | |
| Cheddar Cheese | 0.40 |

| **Vegetables and Pulses** | |
|---|---|
| Haricot beans (boiled) | 2.5 |
| Mung beans (raw) | 8.0 |
| Red kidney beans | 6.7 |
| Avocado pear | 1.5 |
| Lentils (boiled) | 2.4 |
| Butter (lima) beans (boiled) | 1.7 |
| Parsley | 8.0 |
| Spring greens (cabbage) (boiled) | 1.3 |
| Leeks (boiled) | 2.0 |

| **Fruit** | |
|---|---|
| Apricots | 0.4 |
| Bananas | 0.4 |
| Blackberries | 0.9 |
| Dates (dried) | 1.6 |
| Figs (dried) | 4.2 |
| Sultanas (golden raisins) (dried) | 1.8 |
| Prunes (dried) | 2.9 |
| Raisins (dried) | 1.6 |
| Strawberries | 0.7 |

*Foods containing vitamin C*

| **Dairy** | |
|---|---|
| Milk fresh whole | 1.5 |
| Natural yogurt | 0.4 |

|  | mg |
|---|---|
| **Vegetables** | |
| Asparagus (boiled) | 20 |
| Runner beans (boiled) | 5 |
| Broad (sava) beans (boiled) | 15 |
| Broccoli tops (boiled) | 34 |
| Brussels sprouts (boiled) | 40 |
| Cabbage red (raw) | 55 |
| Radishes | 25 |
| Spinach (boiled) | 25 |
| Watercress | 60 |
| Cauliflower (boiled) | 20 |
| Spring greens (cabbage) | 30 |
| Avocado pear | 15 |
| Leeks (boiled) | 15 |
| Lettuce | 15 |
| Mustard and cress | 40 |
| Onions (raw) | 10 |
| Spring onions (scallions) (raw) | 25 |
| Parsley | 150 |
| Parsnips (boiled) | 10 |
| Peas fresh (boiled) | 15 |
| Peppers (bell peppers) green (boiled) | 60 |
| Potatoes (baked) | 5–16 |

| **Meat** | |
|---|---|
| Lamb kidney | 9.0 |

| **Fruit (raw unless otherwise stated)** | |
|---|---|
| Apples | 10 |
| Apples (baked with sugar) | 14 |
| Apricots (fresh) | 7 |
| Banana | 10 |
| Blackberries | 20 |
| Blackcurrants | 200 |
| Gooseberries green (stewed) | 31 |
| Grapes (white) | 4 |
| Grapefruit | 40 |
| Guavas (canned) | 180 |
| Lemons (whole) | 80 |

## Fruit (continued)

| | mg |
|---|---|
| Lychees | 40 |
| Oranges | 50 |
| Orange juice (fresh) | 50 |
| Peaches (fresh) | 8 |
| Pears (eating) | 3 |
| Pineapple (fresh) | 25 |
| Plums | 3 |
| Raspberries | 25 |
| Rhubarb (stewed) | 8 |
| Strawberries | 60 |
| Coconut (fresh) | 2 |
| Grapefruit juice (unsweetened) | 28 |

*Note:* Nuts generally have only a trace of vitamin C

*Foods containing vitamin E*

## Oils

| | mg |
|---|---|
| Cod liver oil | 20.0 |
| Sunflower seed oil | 48.7 |
| Peanut oil | 13.0 |
| Olive oil | 5.1 |

## Meat

| | |
|---|---|
| Lamb (cooked) | 0.18 |
| Lamb kidney | 0.41 |
| Pork (cooked) | 0.12 |
| Chicken (roast meat only) | 0.11 |

## Eggs

| | |
|---|---|
| Eggs (boiled/poached) | 1.6 |

## Fish

| | mg |
|---|---|
| Cod (baked) | 0.59 |
| Halibut (grilled) | 0.90 |
| Herring (grilled) | 0.30 |
| Mussels (boiled) | 1.2 |
| Salmon (canned) | 1.5 |
| Tuna (canned in oil) | 6.3 |

## Nuts

| | |
|---|---|
| Almonds | 20.0 |
| Brazils | 6.5 |
| Hazelnuts | 21.0 |
| Peanuts | 8.1 |

## Fruit

| | |
|---|---|
| Blackberries (raw) | 3.5 |
| Blackcurrants | 1.0 |

## Vegetables

| | |
|---|---|
| Asparagus (boiled) | 2.5 |
| Broccoli tops (boiled) | 1.1 |
| Brussels sprouts (boiled) | 0.9 |
| Parsley | 1.8 |
| Spinach (boiled) | 2.0 |
| Avocado | 3.2 |

*Foods containing calcium*

## Cereals

| | |
|---|---|
| Brown flour | 150 |
| Oatmeal (uncooked) | 55 |
| Soya flour | 210 |
| Wholemeal (wholewheat) bread | 23 |
| Brown bread | 100 |
| Muesli | 200 |

## Fish

|  | mg |
|---|---|
| Haddock (fried) | 110 |
| Pilchards (canned in tomato sauce) | 300 |
| Sardines (canned in oil) | 550 |
| Sprats (fried) | 710 |
| Tuna (canned in oil) | 7 |
| Shrimps (boiled) | 320 |
| Whitebait (fried) | 860 |
| Salmon (canned) | 93 |
| Kipper (baked) | 65 |
| Plaice (steamed) | 38 |

## Fruit

| Apricots (dried) | 92 |
|---|---|
| Blackberries (raw) | 63 |
| Figs (dried) | 280 |
| Lemons (whole) | 110 |
| Rhubarb (stewed) | 93 |
| Tangerines | 42 |

## Dairy

| Milk | 120 |
|---|---|
| Milk dried (skimmed/skim) | 1190 |
| Cheddar cheese | 800 |
| Parmesan cheese | 1220 |
| Cottage cheese (ricotta) | 800 |
| Yogurt (natural) | 180 |

## Vegetables and Pulses

| Carrots (raw) | 48 |
|---|---|
| Celery (raw) | 52 |
| Parsley (raw) | 330 |
| Spinach (boiled) | 600 |
| Watercress | 220 |
| Turnips (boiled) | 55 |
| French beans (boiled) | 39 |
| Haricot beans (boiled) | 65 |
| Broccoli tops (boiled) | 61 |
| Spring greens (cabbage) (boiled) | 86 |

## Nuts

|  | mg |
|---|---|
| Almonds | 250 |
| Brazil nuts | 180 |
| Peanuts | 61 |

*Foods containing chromium*

The following foods are known to contain chromium.

### Meat

| Calf liver | 55 |
|---|---|
| Chicken | 15 |
| Lamb chops | 12 |
| Pork chops | 10 |

### Fruit

| Apple | 14 |
|---|---|
| Banana | 10 |
| Orange | 5 |
| Strawberries | 3 |

### Eggs

| Hens' eggs | 16 |
|---|---|

### Fish

| Scallops | 11 |
|---|---|
| Shrimps | 7 |

### Cereals

| Rye bread | 30 |
|---|---|

### Dairy

| Milk | 1 |
|---|---|
| Butter | 13 |

### Vegetables

| Cabbage | 4 |
|---|---|
| Carrots | 9 |
| Fresh chilli | 30 |
| Green beans | 4 |
| Green (bell) peppers | 19 |
| Lettuce | 7 |
| Mushrooms | 4 |
| Parsnips | 13 |
| Potatoes | 24 |
| Spinach | 10 |

### Other

| Brewer's yeast | 112 |
|---|---|

147

*Foods containing polyunsaturated fats*

Certain fish contain essential oils, similar to those found in vegetables. These oils are helpful in maintaining skin quality and may also be of value in preventing pre-menstrual breast tenderness.

Herring
Mackerel
Pilchard
Salmon
Sardines
Sprats
Whitebait

## How to begin

In the next chapter 'A tailor-made nutritional programme' you will find details about charting your symptoms and keeping daily diaries as a record of your progress. I suggest you do the following:

Complete a chart before you begin so that you have a clear picture of your symptoms.

- Follow the specialized diet for a period of three months.

- Keep daily diaries of all your symptoms. These are provided on page 232 at the end of the book.

- Complete another chart after three months. This can then be compared with your first chart to measure your progress.

# 15

# A TAILOR-MADE NUTRITIONAL PROGRAMME – OPTION 3

The tailor-made nutritional programme is designed to help overcome severe symptoms. Having said that, I feel I should also point out that it is a tough programme, and if your symptoms are extremely severe, you may need help initially. If you can't manage to work out your own programme or you feel you need support, you can contact us at the Women's Nutritional Advisory Service.

Before getting too enthusiastic, it's important to understand that 'The Nutritional Programme' involves quite a bit of work. It's not a magic pill or potion that works overnight in your sleep, but an organized regime that requires a substantial amount of will-power to start with.

At the Women's Nutritional Advisory Service we try to work out the best programme for each individual, according to their symptoms and their existing lifestyle. A *realistic* regime stands a good chance of being followed, whereas an idealistic programme that would work wonders in theory is useless if left in a drawer and forgotten about because it's just too difficult to face or follow.

In order to work out each individual's programme, we need a fair amount of information. As I don't have your chart in front of me I can't work out your programme in the usual way. What I *can* do is to set you a series of questions, and then explain to you, according to your answers, how you go about working out your own programme. I will be unveiling some 'trade secrets' in the course of this section of the book, and hopefully most aspects of the Pre-Menstrual Syndrome will have been covered.

## YOUR PERSONAL NUTRITIONAL PROGRAMME

This programme is designed to help moderate and severe sufferers over their symptoms. If you feel your symptoms fit into the definition of moderate or severe on page 152, you would be best advised to follow this more specialized tailor-made nutritional plan. Make a start in completing the chart and the diary provided on pages 154 and 232. Once you are satisfied with your answers, usually after one full cycle, you can begin compiling your own programme.

If you prefer to begin immediately without waiting for the forms to be completed, then I suggest you follow Option 2 – A specialized diet on page 139. Once your precise programme has been formulated you can implement the additional recommendations and make any changes that are needed.

To avoid confusion, remember that recommendations according to your symptoms should be followed in the long term for best results, rather than continuing to follow the general recommendations made in previous chapters. The reason I make this point is that you may find the two sets of instructions conflict in some areas. An example is that the general recommendations suggest eating plenty of whole grains. However we often find that severe symptoms may be aggravated by certain grains and we may therefore suggest that these are omitted from the diet for a specific period of time in some cases. I have covered this in much fuller detail in the section on food allergies on page 163.

## A STEP-BY-STEP GUIDE
## TO WORK OUT YOUR OWN PROGRAMME

### STEP ONE – HOW TO CHART YOUR SYMPTOMS

Begin by completing the first Pre-Menstrual Syndrome Chart on page 154. This should ideally be completed in two parts.

The left-hand column deals with how you feel normally when you are *not* pre-menstrual. *This column should be completed three days after your period has started.*

The right-hand column deals with how you feel pre-menstrually when your symptoms are at their worst. *This column should be completed two days before your period is due.*

In order to work out your score, you must place a tick by each symptom in both columns. Here is an example of a completed chart. You can see how the symptoms become far more severe pre-menstrually (on the right-hand side of the chart).

150

## ANITA WALKER

| SYMPTOMS | WEEK AFTER PERIOD (Fill in 3 days after period) | | | | WEEK BEFORE PERIOD (Fill in 2-3 days before period) | | | |
|---|---|---|---|---|---|---|---|---|
| | None | Mild | Moderate | Severe | None | Mild | Moderate | Severe |
| **PMT - A** | | | | | | | | |
| Nervous Tension | ✓ | | | | | | | ✓ |
| Mood Swings | ✓ | | | | | | | ✓ |
| Irritability | ✓ | | | | | | | ✓ |
| Anxiety | ✓ | | | | | | | ✓ |
| **PMT - H** | | | | | | | | |
| • Weight gain | ✓ | | | | | | | ✓ |
| Swelling of Extremities | | | ✓ | | | | | ✓ |
| Breast Tenderness | ✓ | | | | | | | ✓ |
| Abdominal Bloating | | ✓ | | | | | | ✓ |
| **PMT - C** | | | | | | | | |
| Headache | ✓ | | | | | | ✓ | |
| Craving for Sweets | ✓ | | | | | | | ✓ |
| Increased Appetite | ✓ | | | | | | | ✓ |
| Heart Pounding | ✓ | | | | ✓ | | | |
| Fatigue | ✓ | | | | | | | ✓ |
| Dizziness or Fainting | ✓ | | | | ✓ | | | |
| **PMT - D** | | | | | | | | |
| Depression | ✓ | | | | | | | ✓ |
| Forgetfulness | ✓ | | | | | | | ✓ |
| Crying | ✓ | | | | | | ✓ | |
| Confusion | ✓ | | | | | | | ✓ |
| Insomnia | ✓ | | | | | | | ✓ |
| **OTHER SYMPTOMS** | | | | | | | | |
| Loss of Sexual Interest | ✓ | | | | | ✓ | | |
| Disorientation | ✓ | | | | | | | ✓ |
| Clumsiness | ✓ | | | | | | | ✓ |
| Tremors/Shakes | ✓ | | | | | | | ✓ |
| Thoughts of Suicide | ✓ | | | | | | | ✓ |
| Agoraphobia | ✓ | | | | | | | |
| Increased Physical Activity | ✓ | | | | ✓ | | | |
| Heavy/Aching Legs | ✓ | | | | | | | ✓ |
| Generalized Aches | ✓ | | | | | | | ✓ |
| Bad Breath | ✓ | | | | | | | ✓ |
| Sensitivity to Music/Light | ✓ | | | | ✓ | | | |
| Excessive Thirst | ✓ | | | | | | | ✓ |

Do you have any other PRE-MENSTRUAL SYMPTOMS not listed above?

1. _____

2. _____

3. _____

4. _____

•5.    How much weight do you gain before your period?   7–10 lbs

151

### Severity of symptoms

You will notice that on the chart you are asked to assess whether your symptoms are mild, moderate or severe. Each of these categories has a numerical score as follows:

0 = None.
1 = Mild.
2 = Moderate.
3 = Severe.

### Mild, moderate and severe defined

(1) **Mild**      Means that symptoms are present but they do not interfere with your activities. You feel all right, but are aware that some physical and emotional changes are taking place as your period approaches.

(2) **Moderate**  Means that symptoms are present and they do interfere with some activities, but they are not disabling. You feel well below par and maybe even cancel arrangements. The family would be aware your period is on its way, maybe even before you are.

(3) **Severe**    Means that symptoms are not only present, they interfere with all activities. They are severely disabling and it's likely that life would be pretty hard to cope with until the symptoms pass.

Using Anita's first chart on page 151 as an example, let's go through it section by section so that you can understand how it works.

### PMT A, H, C and D

**PMT A – Anxiety.** In order to 'qualify' for PMT A your score must be 4 or above for this section. To get your final score you subtract the score for the week after your period from the score for the week before your period. Anita scored 0 after her period and 12 pre-menstrually. Therefore, her overall score is 12, so she certainly does qualify for PMT A.

The reason for subtracting one score from another in this fashion is to attempt to get the *actual* pre-menstrual score. For example, if you have moderate regular headaches all month and they become severe pre-menstrually your real pre-menstrual headache score is only 1, as this symptom only moved from mild to moderate. Compare this to another person who usually has no headaches, but has severe pre-menstrual headaches: the pre-menstrual headache score would be 3 here.

Not to subtract the usual situation for the rest of your cycle from the pre-menstrual situation would create a false picture.

This method of scoring applies to all four categories.

**PMT H – Hydration.** For PMT H you also need a score of 4 to qualify. Anita scored 3 after her period and 10 before her period, giving her a total score of 7. She therefore qualifies.

**PMT C – Sugar craving.** For PMT C there are six symptoms. You will need an overall score of 6 to qualify. Anita scored 0 after her period and a score of 11 before her period. Her overall score was therefore 11.

**PMT D – Depression.** And finally for PMT D, a score of 5 is necessary as there are five symptoms listed in this category. Anita scored 0 after her period and 14 pre-menstrually. Her total score here was 14. She qualified with honours!

Once you have completed your chart you can go on to work out your scores using this example.

Each category has been dealt with separately. You may find that only one of the four categories applies to you. However, it is perfectly possible to be suffering from several categories, or in fact all four.

Now fill in your first chart and see how you fare.

You will notice an additional section on the chart. This is made up of other symptoms which have been reported repeatedly by patients.

### Is it really pre-menstrual?

The best way to assess your symptoms in order to confirm that they are pre-menstrual is to keep daily diaries as I mentioned previously. After two or three months you will see a definite pattern emerging which will serve to confirm the diagnosis of PMT. Two diaries have been provided for this purpose beginning on page 232. Please feel free to photocopy the diaries if you wish.

If, after three months, it seems that your scores are low and your symptoms seem to be persisting all month rather than pre-menstrually, then it would be best to have a full medical consultation and physical examination to determine whether there is some other problem.

### Diaries

It is not only a good idea, but essential that you keep daily diaries. In fact, some doctors feel that it is necessary to keep a diary for three months in order to confirm the diagnosis of PMT. There are several reasons for this:

- To keep a check on your symptoms.

SYMPTOMS

| | WEEK AFTER PERIOD (Fill in 3 days after period) | | | | WEEK BEFORE PERIOD (Fill in 2-3 days before period) | | | |
|---|---|---|---|---|---|---|---|---|
| | None | Mild | Moderate | Severe | None | Mild | Moderate | Severe |
| **PMT - A** | | | | | | | | |
| Nervous Tension | | | | | | | | |
| Mood Swings | | | | | | | | |
| Irritability | | | | | | | | |
| Anxiety | | | | | | | | |
| **PMT - H** | | | | | | | | |
| • Weight gain | | | | | | | | |
| Swelling of Extremities | | | | | | | | |
| Breast Tenderness | | | | | | | | |
| Abdominal Bloating | | | | | | | | |
| **PMT - C** | | | | | | | | |
| Headache | | | | | | | | |
| Craving for Sweets | | | | | | | | |
| Increased Appetite | | | | | | | | |
| Heart Pounding | | | | | | | | |
| Fatigue | | | | | | | | |
| Dizziness or Fainting | | | | | | | | |
| **PMT - D** | | | | | | | | |
| Depression | | | | | | | | |
| Forgetfulness | | | | | | | | |
| Crying | | | | | | | | |
| Confusion | | | | | | | | |
| Insomnia | | | | | | | | |
| **OTHER SYMPTOMS** | | | | | | | | |
| Loss of Sexual Interest | | | | | | | | |
| Disorientation | | | | | | | | |
| Clumsiness | | | | | | | | |
| Tremors/Shakes | | | | | | | | |
| Thoughts of Suicide | | | | | | | | |
| Agoraphobia | | | | | | | | |
| Increased Physical Activity | | | | | | | | |
| Heavy/Aching Legs | | | | | | | | |
| Generalized Aches | | | | | | | | |
| Bad Breath | | | | | | | | |
| Sensitivity to Music/Light | | | | | | | | |
| Excessive Thirst | | | | | | | | |

Do you have any other PRE-MENSTRUAL SYMPTOMS not listed above?

1. _____

2. _____

3. _____

4. _____

•5.  How much weight do you gain before your period? _____

# MENSTRUAL SYMPTOMATOLOGY DIARY

Month: January

### GRADING OF MENSES

| 0-none | 3-heavy |
|---|---|
| 1-slight | 4-heavy and clots |
| 2-moderate | |

### GRADING OF SYMPTOMS (COMPLAINTS)

0-none
1-mild-present but does not interfere with activities
2-moderate-present and interferes with activities but not disabling
3-severe-disabling. Unable to function.

| Day of cycle | 1 | 2 | 3 | 4 | 5 | 6 | 7 | 8 | 9 | 10 | 11 | 12 | 13 | 14 | 15 | 16 | 17 | 18 | 19 | 20 | 21 | 22 | 23 | 24 | 25 | 26 | 27 | 28 | 29 |
|---|---|---|---|---|---|---|---|---|---|---|---|---|---|---|---|---|---|---|---|---|---|---|---|---|---|---|---|---|---|
| Date | 13 | 14 | 15 | 16 | 17 | 18 | 19 | 20 | 21 | 22 | 23 | 24 | 25 | 26 | 27 | 28 | 29 | 30 | 31 | 1 | 2 | 3 | 4 | 5 | 6 | 7 | 8 | 9 | 10 |
| Period | 1 | 2 | 3 | 3 | 2 | 1 | 0 | 0 | 0 | 0 | 0 | 0 | 0 | 0 | 0 | 0 | 0 | 0 | 0 | 0 | 0 | 0 | 0 | 0 | 0 | 0 | 0 | 0 | 0 |

**PMT-A**

| | 1 | 2 | 3 | 4 | 5 | 6 | 7 | 8 | 9 | 10 | 11 | 12 | 13 | 14 | 15 | 16 | 17 | 18 | 19 | 20 | 21 | 22 | 23 | 24 | 25 | 26 | 27 | 28 | 29 |
|---|---|---|---|---|---|---|---|---|---|---|---|---|---|---|---|---|---|---|---|---|---|---|---|---|---|---|---|---|---|
| Nervous tension | 1 | 0 | 0 | 0 | 0 | 0 | 0 | 0 | 0 | 0 | 0 | 0 | 0 | 0 | 0 | 0 | 0 | 0 | 0 | 1 | 0 | 1 | 1 | 2 | 2 | 3 | 3 | 3 | 2 |
| Mood swings | 0 | 0 | 0 | 0 | 0 | 0 | 0 | 0 | 0 | 0 | 0 | 0 | 0 | 0 | 0 | 0 | 0 | 0 | 1 | 2 | 1 | 2 | 2 | 3 | 2 | 3 | 2 | 2 | 3 |
| Irritability | 0 | 0 | 0 | 0 | 0 | 0 | 0 | 0 | 0 | 0 | 0 | 0 | 0 | 0 | 0 | 0 | 0 | 0 | 0 | 1 | 1 | 2 | 2 | 2 | 2 | 2 | 3 | 3 | 3 |
| Anxiety | 0 | 0 | 0 | 0 | 0 | 0 | 0 | 0 | 0 | 0 | 0 | 0 | 0 | 0 | 0 | 0 | 1 | 1 | 0 | 0 | 0 | 2 | 3 | 3 | 2 | 2 | 2 | 3 | 2 |

**PMT-H**

| | 1 | 2 | 3 | 4 | 5 | 6 | 7 | 8 | 9 | 10 | 11 | 12 | 13 | 14 | 15 | 16 | 17 | 18 | 19 | 20 | 21 | 22 | 23 | 24 | 25 | 26 | 27 | 28 | 29 |
|---|---|---|---|---|---|---|---|---|---|---|---|---|---|---|---|---|---|---|---|---|---|---|---|---|---|---|---|---|---|
| Weight gain | 0 | 0 | 0 | 0 | 0 | 0 | 0 | 0 | 0 | 0 | 0 | 0 | 0 | 0 | 0 | 0 | 0 | 0 | 1 | 1 | 1 | 2 | 2 | 2 | 3 | 2 | 2 | 3 | 3 |
| Swelling of extremities | 0 | 0 | 0 | 0 | 0 | 0 | 0 | 0 | 0 | 0 | 0 | 0 | 0 | 0 | 0 | 0 | 0 | 0 | 0 | 0 | 1 | 1 | 1 | 1 | 2 | 2 | 2 | 2 | 2 |
| Breast tenderness | 0 | 0 | 0 | 0 | 0 | 0 | 0 | 0 | 0 | 0 | 0 | 0 | 0 | 0 | 0 | 0 | 0 | 0 | 0 | 1 | 1 | 1 | 1 | 2 | 2 | 2 | 2 | 2 | 2 |
| Abdominal bloating | 1 | 0 | 0 | 0 | 0 | 0 | 0 | 0 | 0 | 0 | 0 | 0 | 0 | 0 | 0 | 0 | 0 | 1 | 1 | 2 | 2 | 2 | 1 | 2 | 1 | 1 | 2 | 2 | 2 |

**PMT-C**

| | 1 | 2 | 3 | 4 | 5 | 6 | 7 | 8 | 9 | 10 | 11 | 12 | 13 | 14 | 15 | 16 | 17 | 18 | 19 | 20 | 21 | 22 | 23 | 24 | 25 | 26 | 27 | 28 | 29 |
|---|---|---|---|---|---|---|---|---|---|---|---|---|---|---|---|---|---|---|---|---|---|---|---|---|---|---|---|---|---|
| Headache | 0 | 0 | 0 | 1 | 0 | 0 | 0 | 0 | 0 | 0 | 0 | 0 | 0 | 0 | 0 | 0 | 0 | 0 | 0 | 0 | 0 | 0 | 0 | 0 | 0 | 2 | 0 | 0 | 1 |
| Craving for sweets | 0 | 0 | 0 | 0 | 0 | 0 | 0 | 0 | 0 | 0 | 0 | 0 | 0 | 0 | 0 | 0 | 1 | 2 | 2 | 0 | 1 | 2 | 3 | 3 | 3 | 2 | 1 | 2 | 2 |
| Increased appetite | 0 | 0 | 0 | 0 | 0 | 0 | 0 | 0 | 0 | 0 | 0 | 0 | 0 | 0 | 0 | 0 | 3 | 2 | 2 | 1 | 0 | 0 | 2 | 2 | 2 | 2 | 2 | 2 | 2 |
| Heart pounding | 0 | 0 | 0 | 0 | 0 | 0 | 0 | 0 | 0 | 0 | 0 | 0 | 0 | 0 | 0 | 0 | 0 | 0 | 0 | 0 | 0 | 0 | 0 | 0 | 0 | 0 | 0 | 0 | 0 |
| Fatigue | 1 | 1 | 2 | 1 | 0 | 0 | 0 | 0 | 0 | 0 | 0 | 0 | 0 | 0 | 0 | 0 | 0 | 0 | 0 | 0 | 2 | 2 | 3 | 3 | 3 | 3 | 3 | 3 | 3 |
| Dizziness or faintness | 1 | 0 | 0 | 0 | 0 | 0 | 0 | 0 | 0 | 0 | 0 | 0 | 0 | 0 | 0 | 0 | 0 | 0 | 0 | 0 | 0 | 0 | 0 | 0 | 0 | 0 | 0 | 0 | 0 |

**PMT-D**

| | 1 | 2 | 3 | 4 | 5 | 6 | 7 | 8 | 9 | 10 | 11 | 12 | 13 | 14 | 15 | 16 | 17 | 18 | 19 | 20 | 21 | 22 | 23 | 24 | 25 | 26 | 27 | 28 | 29 |
|---|---|---|---|---|---|---|---|---|---|---|---|---|---|---|---|---|---|---|---|---|---|---|---|---|---|---|---|---|---|
| Depression | 1 | 0 | 0 | 0 | 0 | 0 | 0 | 0 | 0 | 0 | 0 | 0 | 0 | 0 | 0 | 0 | 0 | 0 | 1 | 1 | 1 | 2 | 2 | 2 | 3 | 3 | 3 | 3 | 3 |
| Forgetfulness | 0 | 0 | 0 | 0 | 0 | 0 | 0 | 0 | 0 | 0 | 0 | 0 | 0 | 0 | 0 | 0 | 1 | 0 | 3 | 2 | 3 | 3 | 3 | 3 | 3 | 3 | 2 | 2 | 3 |
| Crying | 0 | 0 | 0 | 0 | 0 | 0 | 0 | 0 | 0 | 0 | 0 | 0 | 0 | 0 | 0 | 0 | 1 | 0 | 1 | 2 | 1 | 2 | 3 | 3 | 3 | 3 | 2 | 3 | 3 |
| Confusion | 1 | 0 | 0 | 0 | 0 | 0 | 0 | 0 | 0 | 0 | 0 | 0 | 0 | 0 | 0 | 0 | 0 | 1 | 2 | 2 | 2 | 2 | 2 | 3 | 3 | 2 | 2 | 2 | 2 |
| Insomnia | 1 | 1 | 0 | 0 | 0 | 0 | 0 | 0 | 0 | 0 | 0 | 0 | 0 | 0 | 0 | 0 | 1 | 1 | 1 | 1 | 1 | 2 | 2 | 2 | 1 | 3 | 3 | 3 | 3 |

**PAIN**

| | | | | | | | | | | | | | | | | | | | | | | | | | | | | | |
|---|---|---|---|---|---|---|---|---|---|---|---|---|---|---|---|---|---|---|---|---|---|---|---|---|---|---|---|---|---|
| Cramps (low abdominal) | | | | | | | | | | | | | | | | | | | | | | | | | | | | | |
| Backache | | | | | | | | | | | | | | | | | | | | | | | | | | | | | |
| General aches/pains | | | | | | | | | | | | | | | | | | | | | | | | | | | | | |

NOTES:

- To confirm that you have PMT.

- To show a pattern of when the symptoms occur each month.

- To have as a record so that you can judge whether improvement is occurring, without having to rely on your memory.

The form we use is called the Menstrual Symptomatology Diary (MSD) (see Appendix 8), and was designed by Dr Abraham to enable sufferers to keep an ongoing record of their symptoms. The diary should be filled in at the end of each day, throughout the cycle. There are a few things to remember:

**The first day of your cycle is the day your period begins.** Whether your period comes every 22 days or 32 days is irrelevant here. The day bleeding begins, you start a new diary calling this *Day 1*.

There is an example of a completed diary on page 155.

Now you should start filling in the diary and continue to fill it in at the end of each day.

After a few months you should see a very definite pattern emerging. The most likely pattern is for you to experience few symptoms once your period has arrived until at least ovulation, that is, mid cycle. So you will fill in only noughts in the diary. If you have any symptoms at ovulation, indicate them vertically, according to their severity. As your period approaches, the number you fill in will probably get higher, at least for the symptoms that bother you.


## STEP TWO – PLANNING YOUR DIET

### Making changes

Unfortunately there seems to be some truth in the saying 'old habits die hard'. If you set out bearing this in mind you won't get disillusioned along the way. Following the programme usually involves making quite a few changes in both diet and lifestyle. To be realistic, it does take a while to adjust fully. The first month is usually the most rocky. The new routine may cause a bit of confusion here and there at first and a few surprises along the way. If it seems difficult, remember, it is important to persist until you are out of the woods.


### Forewarned is forearmed

Withdrawal symptoms may occur during the first few days on the programme, and can sometimes last for as long as two weeks. Whilst you shouldn't definitely expect these, it's worth bearing in mind that they are very common. Depriving the body of things which it has grown used to sometimes causes it to 'bite back'. It may seem a strange concept that this should occur as a result of dietary changes. However, it is fairly similar to the mechanism of withdrawing from drugs or alcohol. Due to the possible withdrawal symptoms from certain foods and drinks, it is better not to begin this diet in your pre-menstrual phase. Make a start after your period has arrived.

Giving up tea and coffee, for example, may trigger off a number of changes in the body. These may cause you to feel tired or uptight, anxious and on edge. Headaches may occur and, more often, the desire to eat seems to persist. You will be pleased to hear that all this tends to settle down within days, certainly within a couple of weeks. Once you have passed this stage, if it happens to you at all, life becomes much easier, and before long you will notice new habit patterns forming. So much so that patients often prefer *not* to return to their former habits, simply because their tastes have changed! For example, they lose their desire for salty food and regular cups of strong coffee.

The general consensus of opinion is that it is worth persevering, for there is a light at the end of the tunnel. Our research proves this conclusively. When the Women's Nutritional Advisory Service had been in existence for one year we decided it would be desirable to get some scientific feedback on our results. We looked at the results of a group of women who had been on the programme. They had made dietary changes, taken nutritional supplements and regularly exercised. After three months 89 per cent of the women reported that they felt significantly better and there was a 91 per cent reduction in severe symptoms.

We are also reminded that our efforts are worthwhile by the constant flow of grateful letters we receive from patients. From reading the case histories in Part One you will have had a taste of the magnitude of the original problems and then read about incredible changes that took place. The letters we receive from women who have completed the programme often read like fairy stories. It is no wonder we are keen to see the natural approach to curing PMT being widely used!

If I haven't put you off – let's get down to it! We'll deal with dietary aspects first of all, then supplement recommendations. Just a word before we begin: it is not advisable to start following your programme during your PMT week. The reason for this is that the body can be put under strain initially when making dietary changes and it is not a good idea to have to cope with this pre-menstrually.

First of all, decide from your chart which are your main pre-menstrual symptoms. Refer to the section 'PMT and Other Related Symptoms' on page 139 and decide which vitamins and minerals you should be concentrating on in particular. Then read through the food lists on page 142 to familiarize yourself with the foods high in the relevant nutrient. If you are suffering severely, it's likely to encompass most of the food groups.

## LET'S PUT YOU UNDER THE MICROSCOPE

Some of your symptoms fall into categories which you have now been able to identify, but for severe PMT sufferers there are often other factors which play a major part in their condition. In order to determine whether any of these factors apply to you personally, you will need to examine several groups of symptoms. I have put certain symptoms into groups to make this simpler.

On this page there is a skeleton chart for you to complete as you go along. As you read through the sections that follow, make a note of each recommendation which you feel applies to you. By the time you have finished reading the whole of Part Three of this book you should have your programme noted down for easy reference. A copy of this can be pinned up in your kitchen to remind you of the Dos and Don'ts.

### PERSONAL NUTRITIONAL PROGRAMME
### SUMMARY OF RECOMMENDATIONS

**Diet section**

1.

2.

3.

4.

5.

6.

7.

8.

9.

10.

**Supplement section**

1.

2.

3.

4.

5.

## GENERAL RECOMMENDATIONS

There are general recommendations that should be implemented by all severe sufferers, almost regardless of which categories of PMT they suffer from. The fact that you need to cut out certain food groups now does not mean this will remain so for ever. It is simply a way of giving your body a rest and allowing it to recover. I will explain later how to go about re-introducing some of the foods into your diet.

### 1. Cut out caffeine

Caffeine is addictive, although we do not readily believe it to be so. It is present in tea, coffee, chocolate and cola-based drinks.

Caffeine and some other similar substances tend to aggravate PMT A symptoms, i.e. anxiety, irritability, mood swings and nervous tension. It also affects breast symptoms, and the PMT D symptoms of depression and insomnia.

It is advisable to cut caffeine out completely, and to consume only small amounts of decaffeinated coffee, as this contains other chemicals which may have an effect on PMT symptoms. Fortunately, there are many pleasant alternatives which you will find in healthfood shops.

- There are many varieties of herb tea, some fruity and some more herby in taste, most of which are caffeine-free. The most 'tea-like' substitute we have found is 'Redbush' or 'Rooibosch' tea. This can be made with or without milk. Many former tea addicts have found that after a week or two it tastes far more pleasant than ordinary tea. You will need to shop around and experiment to find teas that suit your palate.

- Dandelion coffee is certainly worth a try. It comes in instant form and in roasted root form. I like to use the root, which I put through my coffee filter.

- There are numerous other cereal alternatives you could try, all of which you should find in a good healthfood shop.

### 2. Reduce your dairy produce consumption

Milk, cheese, cream and yogurt tend to make PMT symptoms far worse, particularly PMT A symptoms. Keep your total daily dairy consumption down to the equivalent of one glass of milk per day. If you have a portion of cheese or a yogurt, bear in mind you have very little milk left from your allowance. There are many non-dairy sources of calcium, which you will find mentioned on the calcium food list. So there is no fear of becoming calcium-deficient.

159

## 3. Keep your salt intake to a minimum

Salt may play a part in Pre-Menstrual Tension. Either in the cooking or added at the table, salt leads to increased water retention which tends to aggravate many of the PMT symptoms. You should also avoid eating salty foods. A diet low in salt is a good idea for many reasons, as well as being of value in the treatment of some of your symptoms. If you have an irresistible desire for salt, try using a salt substitute high in potassium salt, rather than the commonly available sodium salt. You will find that after you have been avoiding salt for three or four weeks you no longer miss it, and will begin to taste the food itself.

## 4. Keep your sugar intake low

Sugar is an important dietary factor in Pre-Menstrual Tension. Sugar and sweet foods such as cakes, biscuits, cookies, puddings, jam (jelly), soft drinks and ice cream are high in calories (kjs) and low in important vitamins and minerals. It is deficiencies in some of these vitamins and minerals which play such a part in pre-menstrual symptoms, particularly vitamin B6 and magnesium. Having a lot of sugar in your diet may also contribute significantly to fluid retention and therefore should be avoided.

It is not widely appreciated that 'junk food' contains a lot of phosphorus, which is known to block the uptake of certain trace minerals. Without these important trace minerals PMT symptoms tend to get worse. By 'junk food' we mean processed food, refined food, prepared food, i.e. packet soups, cakes, etc. and anything that contains added sugar, such as sweets (candy), cakes, biscuits (cookies), chocolates and soft drinks.

Coming off sugar can be difficult. However, there are a number of good alternatives.

- Sweeteners can be used in drinks.

- Low-sugar or sugar-free fruit juice and nut bars can be found in many healthfood shops and used in place of sweets.

- Concentrated apple juice is a good sweetener when cooking. Small amounts of molasses may also be used as it is high in the B vitamins and magnesium.

- There are sugar-free jams (jellies) available in healthfood shops. These are made with fruit and apple juice.

- Watered-down fruit juice is a good substitute for soft drinks as it contains no extra sugar or colouring agents etc.

Unfortunately, honey consists mainly of sugar, and only one or two teaspoons should be consumed a day if you can't resist it. Similarly, small amounts of refined sugar – one teaspoon per day – may also be allowed. The same goes for brown sugar, as it has more or less the same effect on your metabolism.

There are specific supplement recommendations for sugar cravings which are mentioned on page 176.

## 5.   Limit your intake of alcohol

As I mentioned in Chapter 11, regular alcohol consumption can have devastating consequences on the body. Alcohol is known to block absorption of certain trace minerals and to knock out B vitamins from the system. Without these you are far more prone to pre-menstrual symptoms. Try not to consume more than two or three alcoholic drinks per week. Fortunately, there are now alcohol-free wines and beers on the market, so you need not refuse a drink.

## 6.   Reduce cigarette smoking

Smoking may affect the levels of certain vitamins, particularly vitamin C, and also aggravate pre-menstrual breast tenderness as well as PMT A symptoms. It is advisable, therefore, that your cigarette consumption be substantially reduced. You may find it easier to cut down on smoking once you have been on the programme for a few weeks. If you don't succeed at first, try again after a month.

## 7.   Eat your greens!

Green leafy vegetables are the major source of some important vitamins and in particular contain the mineral magnesium which plays a substantial part in the correction of pre-menstrual symptoms. It is vital, therefore, that you have a good helping of salad or green leafy vegetables every day. The greens should preferably be lightly cooked in the minimum of water to preserve their vitamin and mineral content. By careful attention to your diet, your need for vitamin and mineral supplements should be reduced.

## 8.   Eat plenty of raw food

Uncooked food is usually far more nutritious than food that has been cooked. In many cooking processes as much as half of the nutrients are lost. Raw food has a much higher fibre content, too. Aim to eat at least one, and preferably two raw meals per day. Eat plenty of salad stuff, fruit and raw vegetables, all of which are easy to prepare and fairly portable, if you are eating away from home. An excellent book to refer to is *Raw Energy* by Leslie and Susannah Kenton which is mentioned on the Recommended Reading List on page 226.

## 9. A note to vegetarians and vegans

Vegetarians who do not eat meat or fish, and vegans who only consume vegetable produce may need to pay particular attention to certain aspects of their diet, so that they do not become nutritionally deficient. Whilst there are many vegetarians who take great care over their diets, there are still too many who try to exist on lettuce leaves and the like. Apart from all the recommendations made so far, vegetarians and vegans should concentrate on the following.

Make sure you have an adequate balance of proteins in your diet.

No single vegetarian protein contains all the appropriate nutrients required, so it's important to combine the different types of vegetable proteins in your vegetarian meals. Vegetarian proteins include: nuts, seeds, peas, beans, lentils, whole grains, brown rice, sprouted beans and soya bean products.

Whilst beans are particularly nutritious, they often cause abdominal wind. Soaking them for 24 hours before cooking them and de-husking them may reduce the problem.

## 10. Iron and Zinc

Ensure you have an adequate intake of the minerals iron and zinc. You can check on this by referring to the iron and zinc food lists on pages 143 and 144.

## MORE SPECIALIZED PROBLEMS: SECTIONS 1–8

I have split this section up into symptom groups. After reading through the group of symptoms, there are recommendations. If these symptoms apply to you, make a note of the recommendation on your personal chart. If the symptoms don't apply to you, then simply pass on to the next section.

Do you suffer with any of the following? (tick applicable boxes)

| Abdominal bloating | ☐ | Depression | ☐ |
| Excessive wind | ☐ | Mouth ulcers | ☐ |
| Constipation | ☐ | Fatigue | ☐ |
| Diarrhoea | ☐ | | |

If you ticked any two of these symptoms it would be *desirable* for you to follow these recommendations.

If, however, you ticked three or more it is *advisable* for you to read through the recommendations carefully, mark them on your chart, and apply them.

## SECTION 1: SENSITIVITY TO GRAINS

There is evidence to show that the symptoms mentioned above may be linked to food allergy, in particular to wheat, oats, barley, rye and corn. We have noticed that a large number of PMT sufferers have had their symptoms made worse because of a sensitivity to one or more grains. I therefore suggest that for the time being you cut out of your diet all the grains mentioned above.

### Assessing for grain sensitivity

You will need to become a nutritional detective by doing the following:

- Stop eating all the above mentioned grains for one month. You can eat one slice of French bread per day if you are desperate! But it's better to try to manage on rice crackers or rice cakes instead. This may seem strange as refined bread is nowhere near as nutritious as wholemeal bread. However, during the refining process most of the grain has been removed and therefore the degree of aggravation caused by this is far less than by a wholegrain loaf.

- After a month, or longer, when you feel that your symptoms have diminished, try introducing the various grains one by one to your diet. Begin just after a period, so that you don't confuse any reaction with PMT symptoms. Choose one grain, e.g. oats. Introduce this into your diet and eat this for several days. If you have no reaction after five days, choose another grain and repeat this process. *DO NOT MIX the grains initially* because if you do get a reaction you won't know exactly what you have reacted to! Continue to do this with all the grains, providing you don't have reactions to any one of them.

### What to do if you have a reaction

The reactions may include diarrhoea or constipation, excessive wind, abdominal bloating, headaches, weight gain, fatigue, confusion, depression, mouth ulcers, rash, irritability and palpitations.

1. Once you have established what you have reacted to, make a note of it and avoid eating this food at all for now. This doesn't mean that you won't be able to eat this food again ever, but it is best avoided for now.

2. Wait until things have settled down again and then try again with another grain.

I appreciate that cutting out all grains is a severe measure. I suggest you begin by just cutting out wholewheat products. You will need to do this for at least four to

163

six weeks to see whether there is any improvement. You can remain on small amounts of white or French bread.

## Constipation

If constipation is a particular problem you might like to try taking some linseed. You can find some very palatable forms of it at your healthfood shop such as Linusit Gold. It is pleasant to eat and can easily be included in your breakfast cereals or salad.

## Foods containing grains

It's surprising how many foods contain grains. Before I began 'label reading' I would never have believed the extent to which grains are used. It's a good exercise to go around the supermarket, reading labels on packets to get an idea of this for yourself. Sometimes labels aren't as explicit as they might be and they just contain the words 'edible starch'. This has to be regarded with suspicion if you are on a grain-free diet. Labelling of food in healthfood shops is usually more reliable and precise.

**Wheat.** The most obvious foods containing wheat are bread, biscuits, cakes and flour made from wheat etc., but wheat is often present in prepared sauces, soups, and processed foods in general. Gluten-free products are not particularly recommended on a wheat-free diet as some of them still contain wheat.

   The following list will give you a rough idea of what to look out for, but I suggest you make a practice of reading labels thoroughly before buying anything.

- Bread, particularly wholemeal, wheatmeal, etc. as these contain more of the natural wheat.

- Cakes, biscuits, pasta, spaghetti, macaroni etc. – pastry, pies, buns, bran (except rice or soya bran), and many breakfast cereals and sausages.

**Oats.** Porridge, oat cookies and oat flakes.

**Rye.** Rye bread (which may also contain wheat), Ryvita.

**Barley.** Often found in packet/tinned soups and stews, barley beverages.

**Corn.** Corn on the cob, corn starch, cornflour, corn (maize), oil and popcorn.

## What to eat instead

There are many substitutes that can be used. You will need to shop around and experiment a little to find the alternatives you prefer. Once you have the hang of it you can cook reasonably normal menus using the substitutes.

**Flour.** You can use rice flour, potato flour, buckwheat flour, millet flour or soya flour. I find a combination of rice flour, which is light, and buckwheat flour, which is rather heavy, works quite well for pastry cases for quiches and for pancakes. (Buckwheat is in fact part of the rhubarb family and is not related to wheat as its name implies.)

I must admit I have not managed to make bread successfully using these alternatives, but would be delighted to hear from anyone who has!

There are many lovely recipe books available with further ideas listed in the Recommended Reading section on page 226.

I have prepared some sample menus to give you an idea of the scope possible. There are also a few recipes included in the recipe section on page 179 as a guideline.

## GRAIN FREE ALLERGY DIET

B = Breakfast   L = Lunch   D = Dinner   S = Sweet

For recipes, see Chapter 16, p 179.

### DAY 1

B   Orange juice
    Buckwheat pancakes (crêpes)
    Dried fruit conserve

L   Fresh avocado and tomato soup
    Jacket potato with cheese

D   Cold mackerel fillets
    Green salad
    Brown rice salad

S   Baked stuffed apples

### DAY 2

B   ½ grapefruit
    Mushroom omelette

L   Sliced turkey
    Orange and beanshoot salad
    Banana

D   Stir fry vegetables and brown rice

S   Grain-free carrot cake

## DAY 3

B   Apple juice
Orange and apple salad
   with millet flakes and nuts

L   Stuffed tomatoes
Waldorf salad
   (using sunflower seeds and
   nuts)

D   Grilled trout
Green leafy vegetables
Carrots and parsnips
   in herb sauce
   (thickened with potato flour)
Boiled potatoes

S   Banana cream

## DAY 4

B   ½ grapefruit
Hot fruit breakfast

L   Tuna omelette
Salad

D   Rosemary and garlic lamb
Brown rice
Jacket potato
   garnished with (bell) peppers
   and parsley

S   Slice of apple cake

## DAY 5

B   Orange juice
Buckwheat pancakes (crêpes)
   with tomatoes, (bell) pepper
   and herbs

L   Leek soup
Jacket potato with prawns
   (shrimps)
Plums

D   Roast chicken
Leaf greens
Carrots
Sprouts and turnips
Boiled potatoes

S   Dried fruit compote and yogurt

## DAY 6

B   ½ grapefruit
Smoked haddock
Mushrooms, tomatoes

L   Green salad
Rice salad and dressing
Apple

D   Liver and onions
Green vegetables
Sauté potatoes

S   Fruity cakes

## DAY 7

B   Oat bran cereal
Orange juice

L   Savory buckwheat pancakes
   (crêpes) with
   salmon, tuna or mackerel
   filling

D   Colourful lentils
   and salad

S   Fruit jelly

### Snacks

With attention focused very much on food, you may get the 'munchies' for a few weeks. There are a number of things to eat between meals which will prevent you from dipping into the cookie jar!

1. Rice crackers or rice cakes from the healthfood shop. The crackers are particularly nice spread with peanut butter, sesame spread or sugar-free jam (jelly), all these from healthfood shops, too.

2. Sesame seeds or other seeds from healthfood shops are pleasant to nibble between meals.

3. Unsalted nuts can be eaten freely, but limit intake of peanuts, which are somewhat indigestible.

4. Fruit of your choice.

5. Rice biscuits or sesame biscuits and healthfood bars that don't contain wheat. Watch out for the sugar, though!


## SECTION 2: SENSITIVITY TO YEAST

Do you suffer from any of the following symptoms?

| | |
|---|---|
| Thrush (more than two episodes in the last five years) ☐ | Cracking at the corners of your mouth ☐ |
| Itchy bottom ☐ | Depression ☐ |
| Bloated abdomen ☐ | Excessive wind ☐ |
| | Cystitis ☐ |

Two or more episodes of thrush and/or any other two symptoms certainly qualify you for the yeast-free diet.


### Yeast sensitivity

Yeast problems in the gut are very common it seems, and they can produce or aggravate a wide variety of symptoms. Everyone has the yeast bug in their gut in harmless quantities (*candida albicans*), but in many people it gets triggered into rapid growth, producing toxins which then affect us, often without our realizing.

A few of the symptoms are of the emotional, mental and physical variety. These are also often 'allergic' type symptoms.

The more obvious yeast conditions are thrush in the vagina or in the mouth, cystitis, abdominal bloating and flatulence.

Many PMT symptoms seem to be aggravated by the yeast bug, *candida*. The vague symptoms of confusion, fatigue, lethargy, depression, poor memory, the feeling of 'not really being there' etc. – the list seems endless.

There are several actions that can be taken to prevent this problem continuing.

### Avoiding yeast in food

It is surprising how many foods contain yeast. Yeast is used frequently in food preparation processes, in which case it is generally marked on the label of the product. However, yeast is a fungus which grows on food, particularly left-over food, even if well covered. It is also particularly fond of foods with an acid-base like citrus fruits and vinegar.

The following list is a guide to foods high in yeast, which you should try to avoid if you want to reduce the PMT symptoms mentioned above.

1. All foods containing sugar or honey, as yeast thrives on sugary or starchy food.

2. All bread, buns, biscuits, cakes etc.

3. Most alcoholic drinks often depend on yeasts to produce the alcohol, especially beer.

4. Citrus fruit juices – only fresh home-squeezed juice is yeast-free.

5. Malted cereals, malted drinks.

6. Pickles, sauerkraut, olives, chilli peppers.

7. Blue cheese (Roquefort).

8. Mushrooms and mushroom sauce.

9. Hamburgers, sausages and cooked meats made with bread or breadcrumbs. Yeast extract (Miso).

10. All fermented foods.

11. Dried fruits.

12. Left-over or stale food.

13. Vitamins. All B-vitamin preparations are likely to be derived from yeast unless otherwise stated; but most manufacturers do make some B-vitamin preparations which are free of yeasts.

## Other contributory factors

Apart from dietary changes there are a few other areas to check. The Pill can make yeast problems worse and should be avoided. Advice should be sought from the Family Planning Clinic for an alternative method of contraception. If the symptoms persist you may need to consult your doctor.

## Hints for beating thrush

- Wear cotton underwear instead of nylon.

- Douche with live yogurt for immediate relief.

- Get your sexual partner treated as well, as it is highly likely that you would pass it back and forwards to each other.

There are some very helpful books on the subject of yeast problems on page 226.

# ANITA'S THRUSH PROBLEMS

'I had continual thrush. I had been under my doctor for this problem and we had tried everything but nothing handled it. I had oral tablets, pessaries to insert in the vagina, creams etc. I tried using live yogurt and even baby oil; I changed my underwear and even stopped wearing tights. Nothing made an impression on the thrush until it was suggested that my diet was continually aggravating the thrush and I went on the nutritional programme. I was asked to stick to the recommendations strictly and my thrush cleared up completely. Wheat does make a difference to me. I'm okay now if I have one or two slices of bread or a small amount of cereal, but if I go beyond that I'll start to bloat. The minute I had a little alcohol as well back would come my thrush. So when I get the feeling I'm going to develop it, I cut out all foods containing yeast. I used to be absolutely plagued with thrush. It has totally vanished now, I haven't had any re-occurrence for at least 18 months.'

# GERALDINE'S THRUSH PROBLEMS

'I had thrush all the time before I went on the programme. The hospital gave me a prescription and told me to use it for three months and not to have any sexual contact with my husband whatsoever in the meantime! Our marriage was already going through a very rough phase at this point, and I'd already tried this treatment before. I tried using the treatment again. It helped for a bit, but as soon as I stopped it the thrush was worse than ever. I had more pessaries and even went into hospital where it was suggested I paint the affected area violet. Diet certainly *did help. Once I cut out sugary foods and other yeast-based foods it made a tremendous difference and the thrush began to clear up by itself.'*

## SECTION 3: HEADACHES

Do you suffer from the following?

Migraine headaches? ☐

Regular pre-menstrual headaches? ☐

**Migraine symptoms** may be aggravated by cheese, alcohol, oranges, tea, coffee, chocolate, fermented foods, potted foods and pastes, yeast and wholemeal (wholewheat) bread, smoked and preserved food and yeast extract. It is therefore advisable to avoid these foods where possible for at least a period of two to three months to see whether it makes any difference to your symptoms.

Make sure any vitamin supplements you take are yeast-free.

## SECTION 4: SUGAR CRAVINGS

Do you suffer with excessive sugar cravings? There are several things you can do if sugar cravings are a problem.

- Sugar cravings could well improve by taking particular supplements, including vitamin B complex, magnesium and the mineral chromium. Chromium deals with sugar balance in the body, and thus plays an important and effective role in controlling sugar cravings.

- Eat a diet rich in foods containing chromium (see page 147).

- Whilst you are experiencing the sugar cravings, eat little and often. In other words, have five or six smaller meals per day, rather than three larger ones. This will help your blood sugar to remain constant and prevent you from having the extreme sugar cravings.

## SECTION 5: IRON DEFICIENCY

Do you suffer with the following?

Heavy periods ☐    Cracking at the corners of the mouth ☐

Fatigue ☐    A sore tongue ☐

170

Heavy periods alone can cause iron deficiency. The other symptoms mentioned above may serve to confirm this. IUDs can sometimes cause heavy bleeding, so if you have a coil, it might be advisable to have a check-up and possibly consider an alternative method of contraception.

With any of the above symptoms you would be wise to ask your doctor to check your serum iron, to see whether you may need some iron supplements. In the meantime you should concentrate on eating iron-rich foods (see page 144).

## SECTION 6: ZINC DEFICIENCY

Do you suffer with any of the following?

| | | | |
|---|---|---|---|
| Acne | ☐ | Eczema | ☐ |
| White spots on your nails | ☐ | Poor hair growth | ☐ |
| Split brittle nails | ☐ | Infertility | ☐ |

Any combination of the above symptoms may indicate that you need to increase your intake of zinc. This can be done by concentrating on foods rich in zinc and initially by taking a zinc supplement.

## SECTION 7: FATTY ACID DEFICIENCY

Do you have any of the following?

| | | | |
|---|---|---|---|
| Dry rough pimply skin on the upper arms or thighs | ☐ | Dandruff | ☐ |
| Red greasy skin | ☐ | Dry flaky skin | ☐ |
| | | Eczema | ☐ |

These symptoms may indicate that you are short of essential fatty acids. If you feel this may be so, you can refer to the Food List on essential fats on page 148. Evening primrose oil capsules may be helpful, as is cold pressed linseed oil when taken orally.

## SECTION 8: BREAST TENDERNESS

Do you suffer with severe breast tenderness or lumpy breasts pre-menstrually? There are a number of preventive measures you can take:

- Eat a low salt diet.

- Cut out tea and coffee.

- Cut out cigarettes, or at least cut down.

- Restrict your dairy produce intake.

- Keep alcohol consumption to a minimum.

- If taking the contraceptive pill it might be worth changing your Pill or using an alternative method of contraception.

## TAKE ONE STEP AT A TIME

There are many new ideas for you to absorb. If you don't feel you can make the necessary changes all at once, then make them gradually. The closer you follow the recommendations, the better off you are likely to feel after you have overcome any withdrawal symptoms that may occur at the very beginning.

It's quite normal to feel sceptical about the value of making such drastic changes. It is only when you start to feel better that you are likely to believe that this is a workable solution.

## WILL YOU BE ON A RESTRICTED DIET FOR EVER?

There seems to be a definite difference between a 'food allergy' and a 'food sensitivity'. More often than not we find that severe PMT cases are suffering with food sensitivity rather than actual allergy, although there are cases where women are violently allergic to certain types of food.

Realistically, if you are suffering with severe symptoms, you need to give your body a complete rest for a minimum of two to three months. We often find it takes as much as six months to a year before the body is really back to normal, and can once again cope fully with foods that have been eliminated.

If you notice unpleasant side-effects occurring when you begin to reintroduce the grains, one by one, or products containing yeast, discontinue them for another month or two, before attempting to reintroduce them again. Usually, the very fact that there is so much progress occurring is an incentive to continue with the nutritional programme.

Occasionally we have found that some unfortunate souls have what seems to be a permanent allergy to a particular food, which when reintroduced continues to make them feel very unwell. In these cases the women themselves usually decide that it is better to be well and do without the food in question than to suffer unnecessarily.

It is probably better not to reintroduce foods to your diet during your pre-menstrual week. I usually suggest waiting until your period is over and you are feeling at your best.

## CHEATING

One for one, the women who go through the programme cheat at some point. Not only do we expect it, we also think it is a positive step. It's only when you have put the system to the test yourself that you really begin to follow it because you believe in it, rather than following it because someone else said it might work.

I have to smile when I think of the stories I'm told about broken diets. I've been through restricted diets myself, so I know what happens. It goes like this. You begin to feel so well on the diet, in fact you've almost forgotten how rotten you felt initially. Amazing how the memory of pain and discomfort evaporates!

You begin to doubt that you really have food sensitivities, perhaps it's just a coincidence that you felt 'unwell' at the time you were eating your favourite restricted food. So you decide to blow the diet. You eat and enjoy one or two days' helpings of the forbidden 'fruit'. Sometimes the symptoms return within an hour or two, sometimes they creep on within a day or so; either way, you have the symptoms back again and you remember what feeling so unwell was like. You now realize that dietary factors and your symptoms are clearly related. So it's back on the diet with a far more self-determined resolution not to cheat!

## IN THE LONG TERM

Once you have been following the dietary and supplement recommendations closely for three or four months, and you have noticed substantial improvement, you can then start to relax a bit. As long as you follow the basic recommendations most of the time, the occasional indulgence shouldn't hurt. Make sure it's only occasional to begin with, and preferably not in the pre-menstrual week. As a general rule, supplements should not be necessary in the long term. They should be taken until you feel that your symptoms are well under control. This may take as little as three or four months or as long as nine months to a year.

Occasionally, months after completing your programme, symptoms may recur. Times of great stress and general illness may, in some circumstances place extra

173

nutritional demands on your body and this may bring on some of the old symptoms. Should this happen to you, identify which PMT category they fall into and take the appropriate dietary action. Use your original programme to help you.

Again, as symptoms reduce, gradually return to the maintenance recommendations and reduce the supplements gradually. It is important to do this in stages as abrupt withdrawal can often lead to recurrence of symptoms.

Do remember to take action quickly with any symptoms so that they can be relieved quickly.

## STEP 3 – CHOOSING YOUR SUPPLEMENTS

We never advise women to take random supplements without some sort of advice. Our bodies are fairly sensitive mechanisms which have specific needs. Too much of a particular nutrient can cause imbalances and consequently other problems in the long term.

Before considering supplements, have a look at the chart called 'Physical Signs of Vitamin and Mineral Deficiency' on the next page: you might recognize some of the signs of vitamin and mineral deficiency which you have had for years but accepted as being 'normal'.

## PHYSICAL SIGNS OF VITAMIN AND MINERAL DEFICIENCIES

There are several useful supplements that can be tried in conjunction with each other. Assuming your symptoms are fairly severe and you are looking for the most effective treatment I will first suggest the optimum regime to begin on, regardless of cost. I will then go on to discuss cheaper, and finally, still cheaper alternatives. As you decide which supplements to try, make a note of their name and the daily dosage on your personal tailor-made programme.

## MULTI-VITAMIN AND MINERAL SUPPLEMENTS

The first and most basic supplement to take is a multi-vitamin and mineral supplement which contains goodly amounts of the essential nutrients mentioned.

The most tried and tested multi-vitamin and mineral supplement for PMT is an American supplement, formulated by Dr Guy Abraham, Optivite for Women. It has been through several American clinical trials and has been shown to raise progesterone levels. It is available in the USA and the UK.

## PHYSICAL SIGNS OF
## VITAMIN AND MINERAL DEFICIENCY

| Sign or Symptom | Can be Caused by Deficiencies of: |
| --- | --- |
| Cracking at the corners of the mouth | Iron, vitamins B12, B6, Folic acid |
| Recurrent mouth ulcers | Iron, vitamins B12, B6, Folic acid |
| Dry, cracked lips | Vitamin B2 |
| Smooth (sore) tongue | Iron, vitamins B2, B12, Folic acid |
| Enlargement/prominence of taste buds at tip of the tongue (red, sore) | Vitamins B2, or B6 |
| Red, greasy skin on face, especially sides of nose | Vitamins B2, B6, zinc or essential fatty acids |
| Rough, sometimes red, pimply skin on upper arms and thighs | Vitamin B complex, vitamin E or essential fatty acids |
| Skin conditions such as eczema, dry, rough, cracked, peeling skin | Zinc, essential fatty acids |
| Poor hair growth | Iron or zinc |
| Dandruff | Vitamin C, vitamin B6, zinc, essential fatty acids |
| Acne | Zinc |
| Bloodshot, gritty, sensitive eyes | Vitamins A or B2 |
| Night blindness | Vitamin A or zinc |
| Dry eyes | Vitamin A, essential fatty acids |
| Brittle or split nails | Iron, zinc or essential fatty acids |
| White spots on nails | Zinc |
| Pale appearance due to anaemia | Iron, vitamin B12, Folic acid, essential to consult your doctor |

The Women's Nutritional Advisory Service has conducted two trials on Optivite, the results of which are detailed on page 177.

We usually recommend that four tablets be taken per day during the first few months. After this, reduce down to two per day until mid cycle, increasing to four per day during your pre-menstrual time. Sometimes, in severe cases, six tablets should be taken per day. If your symptoms are moderate, then a lower dosage may be used.

There are other multi-vitamin and mineral tablets available. We tend to favour Optivite merely because it has been through so many clinical trials. Other multi-vitamins and minerals that did well in trials were PMZ and Premence 28. In Australia, New Zealand and Singapore there is a supplement called PMT, which is produced by Blackmores Laboratories. This supplement did well in a recent clinical trial and is recommended by the Women's Nutritional Advisory Service.

There are certain situations when other supplements need to be taken alongside your multi-vitamin and mineral tablets, some of these are listed on the next chart.

| Problem | Type of Supplement | Daily Dosage | Available from |
|---|---|---|---|
| PMT A, H, C, D | Optivite | 2–6 tabs per day | Boots, chemists and healthfood shops (UK) Optimox (USA) |
| PMT A, H, C, D | Premence 28 | 1 tab per day | Some chemists and healthfood shops (UK) |
| PMT A, H, C, D | PMZ | 2 tabs per day | Chemists and health-food shops |
| Breast problems | Vitamin E | 400 IUs daily | Healthfood shops |
| Extreme nervous tension, drug withdrawals | Strong vitamin B complex | 1–2 tabs per day drug | Healthfood shops |
| Sugar cravings | Sugar Factor | 1– 2 tabs per day | Nature's Best (mail order) |
| Eczema, urticaria (nettle rash other skin problems) | Evening primrose oil | 4–8×500 mg capsules daily | Boots, chemists and healthfood shops |
| Dry rough skin/ dandruff | Cold pressed linseed oil | 2 tbsp with fruit juice at night | Healthfood shops |
| Period pains/ palpitations or insomnia | Magnesium chelate or magnesium hydroxide mixture | 2×500 mg tabs per day, 15 ml taken as 5 ml, 3 times per day | Healthfood shops and chemists |

## RESULTS OF CLINICAL TRIALS PERFORMED BY THE PRE-MENSTRUAL TENSION ADVISORY SERVICE

| Name and type of product | Available from | Dosage given | Improved a lot | Improved slightly | No worse but no better |
|---|---|---|---|---|---|
| Optivite | Nature's Best | 4 per day increasing to 8 per day pre-menstrually | 71.5% | 16.5% | 12% |
| Optivite | Nature's Best | 2 per day increasing to 4 pre-menstrually | 65% | 31% | 6% |
| Evening primrose oil (Efamol) | Healthfood shops | 8×500 mg capsules per day | 64% | 19% | 17% |
| Premence 28 | Chemists | 1 per day | 72.1% | 18.6% | 9.3% |
| PMT | Australia New Zealand Singapore | 2 per day | 60% | 30% | 10% |

Out of all the supplements available, only Optivite and Efamol have shown consistently significant results in clinical trials. For details of supplements available in Australia and New Zealand see Appendix 4.

## IMPORTANT POINTS

- Never take supplements without the consent of your GP if you have a current medical problem.
- Always begin taking your supplements gradually. For example, if you are due to take two or four per day of a particular supplement, begin taking them one tablet per day and gradually build up to the optimum dosage over the period of a week or two. Take them after meals unless otherwise specified.

### How to cut down on your supplements

- Cut down on the dosage very gradually over a period of months rather than weeks, but keep taking the supplements each day of your cycle.

- Once you have reduced the dosage gradually, if you feel that your symptoms are well under control you can leave the supplements off altogether the week after your period.

- After another couple of months you can remain supplement-free for two weeks after your period.

- You might prefer to keep taking supplements pre-menstrually, or to cut them out completely and only take them at times of great stress. Some women prefer to take small doses daily on a permanent basis. There is no harm in doing so. As you will probably recognize from Chapter 11, which deals with our diet today, the nutrients in our food are often lost to us, therefore taking supplements in the long term as a general health aid may be a sensible move.

## WHAT ABOUT YOUR DRUGS?

If you are currently taking prescribed drugs from your doctor, I don't advise you to stop taking them or reduce them without his or her consent. Having said that, we do find that most women, once established on their nutritional programme, no longer feel the need for their tranquillizers, anti-depressants or sleeping pills.

Vitamins and minerals can be taken quite happily alongside most drugs. There are a few exceptions however. Any antibiotic in the tetracycline family should not be taken with minerals. Evening primrose oil should not be taken by anyone who has a history of epilepsy. When you feel the time has come to reduce your drugs, do go to see your doctor before taking any action, especially if you have been taking the drugs for a long period of time. Coming off drugs suddenly may bring on nasty withdrawal symptoms.

# 16

# NUTRITIOUS
# RECIPES

Although this is not designed to be a recipe book, I felt it would be useful for you to have some guidelines to work with. It's better if you are not short of ideas to begin with: the more you like your new diet, the higher the chances of your sticking to it. In the Recommended Reading List on page 226, I have suggested many inexpensive recipe books which will give you further ideas. It might be an idea to visit a good bookshop and have a browse through the books, so that you can select those you find most suitable.

The recipes I have given cover breakfast, soups, lunch, dinner and sweets. All the recipes are suitable for those of you who are moderate sufferers. For those of you who suffer severely and therefore select a restricted diet, follow the recipes with a code beside them.

### There are two codes:

G = Grain-free.
Y = Low yeast content.
No code = Suitable for all sufferers who are not on restricted diets.

*Note* Imperial and American measures are given in brackets, where appropriate.
Use salt substitute, not salt.
Miso when not in brackets is soya.

## BREAKFASTS

### WHOLEWHEAT PANCAKES (CRÊPES)

*110 g (4 oz/½ cup) wholemeal
(wholewheat or buckwheat) flour
1 small egg*

*300 ml (10 fl oz/1¼ cups) skimmed
(skim) milk
oil for cooking*

Make a thin batter with the flour, egg and skimmed milk, whisking well. Use kitchen paper to wipe a small non-stick frying pan with oil and heat until it is smoking. Pour a generous 2 tablespoons of the batter into the pan and swirl it around to cover bottom as thinly as possible. Cook the batter for 60 seconds, then flip it over with a spatula and cook the other side for a few seconds only. If you are going to eat straight away, tip onto a heated plate – otherwise, stacked pancakes with cling film (plastic wrap) in between can be stored in refrigerator. They can be easily reheated individually on a plate covered with foil over a pan of water, or in the microwave oven.     SERVES 4

### MUESLI

*½ mug (½ cup) dried apricots
½ mug (½ cup) jumbo oats
½ mug (½ cup) barley flakes
¼ mug (¼ cup) large sultanans (golden
raisins)*

*½ pint (1 cup) fresh orange juice
2 apples, grated
milk to mix
¼ mug (¼ cup) chopped mixed nuts
clear honey, to taste*

Put apricots, oats, barley flakes, sultanas and orange juice in a mixing bowl. Cover and leave to soak overnight. Next morning, stir in the apple and sufficient milk to give a soft consistency. Spoon the muesli into dishes and top with chopped nuts and honey.     SERVES 3–4

### HOT FRUITY BREAKFAST

*25 g (1 oz/2 tbsp) lightly crushed millet,
toasted*

*150 ml (¼ pint/½ cup) milk
stewed fruit according to taste*

Mix the millet and milk in a pan. Bring gently to the boil and simmer for 5 minutes, stirring occasionally. Put in a serving bowl, stir in 15–30 ml (1–2 tbsp) stewed fruit, and serve with extra milk substitute or a spoonful of sugar-free jam.     SERVES 1

## DRIED FRUIT CONSERVE   G

200 g (7 oz/1 cup) dried apricots
apple juice

**Use one of the following flavourings**
5 ml (1 tsp) orange flower water

or

5 ml (1 tsp) grated orange peel

or

50 g (2 oz/½ cup) flaked almonds

Soak apricots overnight in water. Put the apricots into a saucepan and just cover them with apple juice, using the minimum amount to ensure a thick purée. Simmer them, uncovered, for about 30 minutes or until they are thoroughly cooked and soft. Cool and then thoroughly blend or sieve them until they have a smooth, thick consistency. Add one of the flavourings.

Purée will keep in refrigerator for about 10 days.    SERVES 2


## SOUPS


## LENTIL AND VEGETABLE SOUP   G

15 g (½ oz) soft vegetable margarine
1 onion, chopped
1 garlic clove, crushed
2 large carrots, finely diced
2 sticks celery, sliced
2 tomatoes, skinned and chopped
50 g (2 oz/1 cup) mushrooms,
   chopped

100 g (4 oz) cabbage, shredded
100 g (4 oz/½ cup) continental lentils,
   pre-soaked
1 litre (1¾ pints) vegetable stock
bouquet garni (sprig parsley, thyme and
   bayleaf tied)
parsley
pepper

Melt margarine in a large saucepan and sauté the onion for five minutes without browning. Add garlic and rest of vegetables and cook gently for five minutes over the heat, then add the stock and bouquet garni, stir in extra parsley and season to taste with pepper.    SERVES 4


## BROCCOLI SOUP   G&Y

225 g (8 oz–1 lb) broccoli, chopped
1.7 litres (3 pints) vegetable stock
1.25 ml (¼ tsp) salt

30 ml (2 tbsp) semi-skimmed (skim)
   milk
pinch nutmeg
pinch cayenne pepper

Combine broccoli, stock and salt in large saucepan, bring to boil. Reduce heat and simmer for 15 minutes. Remove from heat, blend mixture to purée with milk, nutmeg and cayenne. Return to pan, heat through,           do not boil.   SERVE

## NUTTY PARSNIP SOUP   G

25 g (1 oz/1 tbsp) vegetable margarine
1 medium onion, chopped
300 g (10½ oz) parsnips, sliced
1 tbsp smooth peanut butter

dash shoyu (soya derivative, from
  healthfood shops)
1 vegetable stock cube
600 ml (1 pint) water
25 g (1 oz/¼ cup) peanuts, roasted

Melt the margarine in a deep pan. Sauté the onions and parsnips together until beginning to soften. Stir in the peanut butter to coat the vegetables. Add a little shoyu. Bring vegetable stock to the boil and add the water gradually, allowing the peanut butter to thicken slightly. Continue cooking until all ingredients are soft. Blend. Roughly grate the peanuts and scatter on the surface just before serving. (Hazelnuts and hazelnut butter can be used instead.)   SERVES 4

## FRESH AVOCADO AND TOMATO SOUP   G&Y

50 g (2 oz/¼ stick) butter/margarine
1 medium-sized onion, chopped
1 small potato, chopped
450 g (1 lb) tomatoes, quartered
2 garlic cloves

1 bay leaf
30 ml (2 tbsp) tomato purée (paste)
450 ml (¾ pint) vegetable stock
450 ml (¾ pint) milk
2 avocados (ripe)
pepper to taste

Melt the butter/margarine and sauté the onion until transparent. Add potato, tomatoes, garlic, bayleaf, tomato paste and stock. Cover and simmer for 20 minutes. Take off the heat, stirring in the milk and chopped avocado flesh. Remove bay leaf. Blend in small quantities in liquidizer goblet. Adjust seasoning to taste and reheat to serving temperature.   SERVES 4–6

## CHICKEN SOUP   G&Y

1 chicken boned and cut into 2.5 cm
   (1 in) cubes
600 ml (1 pint) water
4 garlic cloves, sliced (optional, to taste)
2 sticks of celery, chopped

2 carrots, chopped
1 medium onion
50 g (2 oz) peas
50 g (2 oz) cooked brown rice
25 g (1 oz) parsley, chopped
herbs and seasoning to taste

Simmer chicken in water for 40 minutes. Add garlic, vegetables and rice and simmer for additional 20 minutes. Serve topped with scissor-snipped fresh parsley. Add herbs according to taste.     SERVES 4

# SALADS

**Always use the very best and freshest ingredients**

## BEANSHOOT SALAD   G&Y

50 g (2 oz/½ cup) almond halves
1 tsp oil
¼ tsp salt

50 g (2 oz) carrots
2 bananas
200 g (8 oz) fresh beanshoots

Put the almonds, oil and salt in small ovenproof dish. Mix well, then roast in the oven at 200°C (400°F/Mark 6) for about 10 minutes until golden. Leave until cold. Grate carrots and slice the bananas, combine with almonds and beanshoots.
    SERVES 4

## WALDORF SALAD   G

4 sticks celery
50 g (2 oz/½ cup) walnuts
1 large dessert apple

150 g (6 oz) Cheddar cheese
salt and pepper
French dressing

Chop the celery and walnuts. Dice the apple and cheese. Mix all the ingredients together in a salad bowl. Add seasoning and dressing to taste.     SERVES 4

## BULGAR AND NUT SALAD

200 g (8 oz/1⅓ cups) bulgar (cracked
 wheat)
1 large sized onion, finely chopped
3 tbsp olive oil
100 ml (4 fl oz) tomato purée (paste)
60 ml (4 tbsp) dried mint

5 ml (1 tsp) ground cumin
5 ml (1 tsp) ground coriander
2.5 ml (½ tsp) ground allspice
110 g (4 oz/1 cup) walnuts and/or
 hazelnuts, very coarsely chopped
juice of 1 lemon

Soak the cracked wheat (available from healthfood shops) in plenty of fresh cold water for 15 minutes, drain it well and squeeze out as much of the water as you can. Fry the chopped onion in a tablespoon of oil until very soft but not yet coloured. Mix all the ingredients in a large serving bowl and leave for about an hour for the bulgar to absorb the flavours and become plump and tender.     SERVES 4

## GRAPEFRUIT AND ORANGE SALAD   G&Y

1 whole grapefruit
1 orange
75 g (3 oz/½ cup) sunflower seeds

50 g (2 oz/½ cup) mixed nuts chopped
orange juice, freshly squeezed

Remove rind of grapefruit and orange and chop flesh, mix with sunflower seeds and nuts and a little orange juice.     SERVES 4

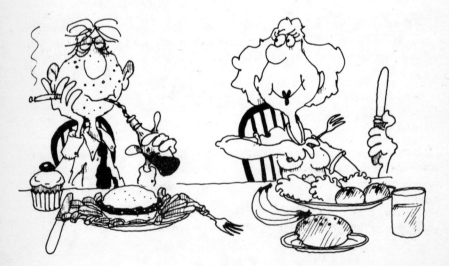

## ORANGE AND CUCUMBER SALAD   G&Y

2 oranges, divided into segments
½ cucumber, thinly sliced

1 small onion, thinly sliced into rings
½ small lettuce

Mix all ingredients together.    SERVES 4


## GREEN BEAN AND SWEETCORN SALAD   Y

200 g (8 oz) young French beans,
  topped and tailed
150 g (6 oz) can sweetcorn

2 spring onions (scallions), thinly sliced
2 tbsp French dressing (not for low yeast
  diet)

Cook the beans in slightly salted boiling water until tender. Drain, refresh in cold running water, leave to cool. Mix together the beans, sweetcorn and onions. Stir together with French dressing.    SERVES 4


## SALAD DRESSINGS


## PEANUT AND CHILLI   G

25 ml (1 fl oz/2 tbsp) peanut oil
1 medium onion, thinly sliced
2.5 ml (½ tsp) chilli powder
5 ml (1 tsp) sugar/honey
5 ml (1 tsp) shoyu/tamari (soy sauce,
  from healthfood shops)
15 ml (1 tbsp) tomato purée (paste)
  (optional)

30–45 ml (2–3 tsbp) peanut butter
  (smooth)
3 cloves garlic, crushed or finely chopped
200 ml (7 fl oz/1 cup) water
200 ml (7 fl oz/1 cup) milk
dash of pepper

Heat oil gently and stir in onion, chilli, sugar/honey and shoyu, cook until onion is soft. Stir in tomato purée, peanut butter and garlic. Add water and milk and bring back to the boil, stirring regularly until mixture is smooth and not too thick. Season with pepper to taste.

It is important that the consistency is not too thick as it will become thick and lumpy if overcooked.    MAKES 2½ CUPS


185

## AVOCADO AND YOGURT DRESSING   G&Y

1 ripe avocado
½ lemon
400 ml (14 fl oz) yogurt

3 cloves garlic (crushed)
pinch of salt and pepper

Halve the avocado and scoop out the flesh, blend or mash immediately with lemon juice. Fold yogurt and garlic into avocado mixture until smooth. Season to taste, or season with chilli or cayenne pepper.   MAKES 2½ CUPS

## YOGURT HERB DRESSING   G

125 ml (5 fl oz/½ cup) natural yogurt
1 clove garlic, crushed
15 ml (1 tbsp) cider vinegar

5 ml (1 tsp) clear honey
15 g (½ oz) parsley
15 g (½ oz) mixed mint and herbs
pinch of salt and pepper

Place all ingredients except herbs in a bowl, adding salt and pepper to taste and mix thoroughly with a fork. Add herbs finely chopped and mix well or blend for 1–2 minutes. Chill until required.   MAKES 1 CUP

## CREAMY TOMATO DRESSING   G&Y

30 ml (2 tbsp) homemade mayonnaise
1 tomato, chopped

10 ml (2 tsp) lemon juice
2.5 ml (½ tsp) dried or 1 tsp fresh basil

Blend all the ingredients together on low speed.   MAKES ABOUT ⅓ CUP

## LUNCHES AND DINNERS

## GRILLED (BROILED) SARDINES   G&Y

Wash and dry sardines, dust with peppered flour (non-wheat flour for restricted diets) and grill (broil) for 5–10 minutes depending on size, turning once.
or
Place sardines on the grill (broiler), sprinkle with pepper and olive oil and grill for 5–10 minutes depending on size, turning once.

## STUFFED PEPPERS   G

1 medium onion
2 sticks celery
100 g (4 oz) mushrooms
1 large tomato
1 medium-sized carrot
25 g (1 oz/½ stick) margarine
100 ml (5 fl oz/½ cup) water
5 ml (1 tsp) tomato purée (paste)

2.5 ml (½ tsp) yeast extract (Miso)
4 medium-size green or red (bell)
   peppers
30 ml (2 tbsp) buckwheat or other grain-
   free flour
seasoning to taste
100 g (4 oz) Cheddar cheese, grated

Chop the onion, celery, mushroom and tomatoes and dice the carrot, melt margarine and fry onion, carrot, celery and mushroom together for 5 minutes. Stir in the tomato, water, tomato purée and yeast extract. Cover and simmer for 10–15 minutes, until just tender. Meanwhile, halve peppers lengthways and remove the seeds, then steam for 10 minutes. Arrange in an ovenproof serving dish. Drain vegetables, reserving the cooking liquid. Fill the peppers with the vegetables. Sprinkle the flour into the vegetable liquid and bring to the boil. Adjust seasoning to taste. Pour over the peppers, sprinkle with the cheese and bake in the oven at 200°C (400°F/Mark 6) for 15 minutes. Serve at once.   SERVES 4

## SPANISH OMELETTE   G&Y

1 small onion, chopped
25 ml (1 fl oz/¼ cup) water
1 stick celery, chopped
1 green (bell) pepper

2 eggs
5 ml (1 tsp) butter
2 tomatoes, chopped
parsley (scissor-snipped)

Place the onions and water in a sealed pan over a medium heat. When water begins to boil reduce the heat to low. Add celery and green pepper and continue cooking until soft. Do not overcook. Beat eggs, melt butter in a medium frying pan over a low heat. Pour in beaten eggs and allow to cook gently. Strain vegetables, tip onto partly cooked omelette and add tomatoes. When cooked serve sprinkled with parsley.   SERVES 1

## STIR FRY VEGETABLES   G†

There are many different combinations of vegetable in season that can be used for stir frying. You can use six or seven different vegetables or only two or three.

To obtain the best results, stir fry vegetables should be cooked with the minimum oil at a high heat as rapid cooking seals in the flavour.

Here are some nice last-minute additions to your stir fry. Experiment to find your favourite seasoning and flavouring. Less well-known ingredients are available from healthfood shops.

### *Seasoning

Salt, pepper, chilli, grated ginger, five spice (use very moderately), sesame seeds (ground), fenugreek (ground), turmeric, coriander, paprika, nori seaweed (toasted and crumbled).

### *Flavouring

Shoyu/tamari, Miso (all Japanese/Chinese condiments made from soya beans), sesame oil, tahini (sesame seed butter), sunflower oil, safflower oil, sherry, vermouth, lemon juice.

*450 g (1 lb) fresh broccoli*
*225 g (8 oz) cauliflower*
*15 ml (1 tbsp) oil*
*2.5 cm (1 in) fresh ginger, sliced and finely shredded*
*2 large carrots, peeled and sliced*

*2.5 ml (½ tsp) sesame oil*
*225 g (8 oz) fresh bean sprouts*
*225 g (8 oz) Chinese leaves or white cabbage, shredded*
*2.5 ml (½ tsp) salt*

Separate the broccoli heads into small florets and peel and slice the stems. Separate the cauliflower florets and slice stems. Heat oil in a large wok or frying pan. When it is moderately hot add ginger shreds. Stir fry for a few seconds. Add the carrots, cauliflower and broccoli and stir fry for 2–3 minutes then add sesame seed oil, bean sprouts and Chinese leaves or white cabbage. Stir fry for further 2–3 minutes. Season to taste. Serve at once.   SERVES 4–6

Ginger can be substituted for garlic and soy sauce can be added in final stage of frying before serving.

† and Y if yeast-free flavouring selected

## MACKEREL WITH HERBS (IN FOIL)   G&Y

4 medium-sized fresh mackerel, gutted
juice of one lemon
freshly ground black pepper

4 small bunches of 4 different fresh
   mixed herbs, e.g. tarragon, chives,
   parsley and sage
little olive oil

Preheat oven to 240°C (475°F/Mark 9). Wash mackerel and sprinkle insides with lemon juice. Add generous sprinkling of pepper. Put bunch of mixed herbs inside each fish and brush skin with oil to avoid sticking, wrap each fish individually in foil, quite tightly, bake for 10–12 minutes and serve.   SERVES 4

## STUFFED MACKEREL IN FOIL

2 large oranges
4 tbsp porridge (rolled oats)
1 medium-sized onion, finely chopped
1 tbsp parsley, finely chopped
1 tbsp raisins

1 apple, grated
pinch of salt
1 tsp dried rosemary or 4 sprigs fresh
   rosemary
4 medium-sized fresh mackerel, gutted

Grate zest of orange, chop flesh into small pieces, discarding pips and any tough pith. Mix the orange zest and flesh with oats, onion, parsley, raisins and grated apple and pinch of salt. Divide mixture into 4 and stuff mackerel loosely. Place rosemary in each fish. Bake in foil as above for about 40 minutes.   SERVES 4

## VEGETARIAN GOULASH   G

45 ml (3 tbsp) oil
1 medium onion, sliced
2 medium carrots, diced
2 medium courgettes (zucchini), sliced
½ small white cabbage, finely shredded
15 ml (1 tbsp) paprika
2.5 ml (½ tsp) caraway seeds

2.5 ml (½ tsp) mixed herbs
pinch of nutmeg
600 ml (1 pint) tomato juice
300 ml (½ pint) water
1 vegetable stock cube
142 ml (¼ pint) soured cream or natural
   yogurt

Heat oil in large saucepan and sauté the onion and carrot until the onion is transparent. Add courgettes and cabbage and cook over medium heat for 10 minutes, stirring frequently. Stir in paprika, caraway seeds, herbs and nutmeg, then add tomato juice, water and stock cube. Cover and simmer for about 20 minutes until the vegetables are just tender. Adjust seasoning with small pinch salt and pepper. Serve each portion with a drop of soured cream or yogurt. Serve at once.   SERVES 4–6

## STEAMED FISH (WITH GARLIC, SPRING ONIONS (SCALLIONS) AND GINGER)   G&Y

350 g (12 oz) firm white fish fillets (cod, sole etc)
2.5 ml (½ tsp) salt
15 ml (1 tbsp) fresh ginger, finely chopped
30 ml (2 tbsp) spring onions (scallions), finely chopped

15 ml (1 tbsp) light soy sauce (not for yeast-free diet)
15 ml (1 tbsp) oil, preferably groundnut
5 ml (1 tsp) sesame oil
2 garlic cloves, peeled and thinly sliced

Rub cleaned and dried fish with salt both sides and leave for 30 minutes. Steam fish over simmering water until just cooked, covering steamer tightly. Sprinkle on the ginger, spring onions and light soy sauce. Heat the two oils together in small saucepan, when hot add garlic slices and brown. Pour the garlic oil mixture over the top of the fish. Serve at once.   SERVES 4

## LAMB PAPRIKA   G

2 onions, sliced
50 g (2 oz) mushrooms, sliced
2 carrots, sliced
4 lamb chops (lean)

30 ml (2 tbsp) paprika
375 ml (¾ pint) water
15 ml (1 tbsp) cornflour (cornstarch) (or alternative grain-free flour)

Mix vegetables together and place in casserole. Arrange chops on top. Stir paprika into water and pour over chops, cover and cook until chops are tender. Remove vegetables and chops and arrange on warm serving dish. Mix cornflour with a little cold water and use to thicken liquid from chops. Cook for 2–3 minutes, pour over chops.   SERVES 2–4

## LIVER WITH ORANGE   G

225 g (8 oz) lamb's liver
30 ml (2 tbsp) wholewheat flour (or alternative grain-free flour)
2.5 ml (½ tsp) dried thyme or basil
25 ml (1½ tbsp) sunflower oil

1 orange, peeled and sliced
grated orange peel
15 ml (1 tbsp) soy sauce
30 ml (2 tbsp) orange juice

Wash liver, slice thinly, pat dry with kitchen paper. Cut out and discard stringy pieces, coat in flour seasoned with herbs. Heat oil in a frying pan and fry liver pieces gently for 5 minutes, turning to cook evenly. Add orange slices and peel, soy sauce and orange juice. Heat through gently and serve.   SERVES 2

## NUT ROAST   G

1 medium onion
25 g (1 oz/¼ stick) butter/margarine
225 g (8 oz/2 cups) mixed nuts
100 g (4 oz/2 cups) cooked brown rice

200 ml (½ pint) vegetable stock
10 ml (2 tsp) yeast extract (Miso)
5 ml (1 tsp) mixed herbs
salt and pepper to taste

Chop onions and sauté in butter until transparent. Grind nuts in a blender or food processor until quite fine. Heat stock and yeast extract to boiling point, then combine all the ingredients including the cooked brown rice together and mix well until the mixture is a fairly slack consistency. Turn into greased shallow baking dish, level the surface, and bake in oven at 180°C (350°F/Mark 4) for 30 minutes until golden brown.   SERVES 4–6

## COLOURFUL LENTILS   G

60 ml (4 tbsp) oil
3 cloves garlic, crushed
4 carrots, chopped
1 green (bell) pepper, chopped
1 red (bell) pepper, chopped
5 ml (1 tsp) basil
3 sticks celery, chopped

15 ml (1 tbsp) brown rice miso
900 ml (1½ pints) hot water
675 g (1½ lb) tomatoes, skinned, seeded
  and chopped
280 g (10 oz) lentils, not presoaked
30 ml (2 tbsp) chopped parsley
seasoning to taste

Heat oil in a pan and add the garlic, carrots, green and red peppers, basil and celery. Cook until the ingredients are soft. Mix the brown rice miso with hot water and add this to mixture, together with the tomatoes. Stir in the lentils. Season to taste. Simmer for 1 hour. Serve, garnished with the chopped parsley.   SERVES 4 OR 6 AS A STARTER

## STUFFING FOR ROAST CHICKEN   G

1 stick celery, finely chopped
2 cloves garlic, crushed
30 ml (2 tbsp) sunflower oil
60 g (2 oz/¼ cup) uncooked long grain
   brown rice
150 ml (¼ pint) hot water

120 g (4 oz/2 cups) mushrooms, sliced
30 g (1 oz/⅙ cup) sultanas
60 g (2 oz/⅓ cup) dried apricots, soaked
   and chopped
30 ml (2 tbsp) tarragon

Fry the celery and garlic in the oil for 2–3 minutes. Add the rice and sauté for a few minutes. Pour in the hot water, stir, then simmer for 5–6 minutes until most of the water has been absorbed, but the rice is still hard. Remove from the heat and mix in the remaining ingredients. Allow to cool for a little, then use to stuff the chicken.

## SWEETS

### FRUIT JELLY   G

22 g (¾ oz) gelatine
600 ml (1 pint) unsweetened fruit juice
   e.g. apple, pineapple

Sprinkle the gelatine on 1 tbsp heated fruit juice and stir well until dissolved. Add the rest of the juice. Put into a wetted mould and chill until set.   SERVES 4

### DRIED FRUIT COMPOTE AND YOGURT   G

15 g (½ oz/1 tbsp) sugar
600 ml (1 pint) water
5–10 cm (2–3 in) stick of cinnamon

450 g (1 lb) mixed dried fruit e.g. apple
   rings, peaches, apricots, prunes, pears
   and sultanas

Dissolve the sugar in the water over a gentle heat, add the cinnamon. Place the dried fruit in a bowl and pour the syrup over. Cover and leave to soak overnight. If the soaked fruit is not tender, replace in the pan and simmer for a few minutes. Serve cold with yogurt.   SERVES 4–6

## RHUBARB FOOL   G&Y

25 g (1 oz/¼ stick) margarine
225 g (8 oz) rhubarb

12–25 g (½–1 oz) brown sugar
200 ml (7 fl oz) natural yogurt

Melt margarine in a pan. Add rhubarb and sugar and cook until tender. Purée rhubarb and yogurt together in a blender. Chill before serving.   SERVES 4

## STUFFED BAKED APPLES   G

4 good-sized cooking apples
1 tbsp honey/sugar-free jam

**Stuffing suggestions**
Dates, cinnamon, raisins and honey

Core apples and slit skins in a ring round the middle. Stuff with chosen filling and honey. Bake until fruit is tender. Serve hot or cold.   SERVES 4

## CARROT CAKE   G

4 eggs
225 g (8 oz/1 cup) caster (superfine)
   sugar
grated rind of 1 lemon

225 g (8 oz/2 cups) ground almonds
225 g (8 oz) carrots, finely grated
25 ml (1½ tbsp) rice flour
5 ml (1 tsp) wheat-free baking powder

Preheat the oven to 180°C (350°F/Mark 4). Separate the eggs. Place yolks, sugar and lemon rind in a bowl or in a blender or food processor and beat together well. Add the almonds and carrots to this mixture. Stir well. Sift the flour and baking powder together then fold into mixture. In another bowl beat the egg whites until they are stiff, then fold them into the mixture. Grease an oblong baking tray 8×12×2 inches (20×30×5 cm). Spread the mixture out in the tray and bake for 45 minutes. Leave to cool in the tray, then cut into slices.   MAKES 10 SLICES

## BANANA CREAM   G

4 medium bananas
15 ml (1 tbsp) lemon juice

400 ml (15 fl oz/2 cups) yogurt
5 ml (1 tsp) honey

Place all ingredients in the blender and blend until creamy. Chill well before serving.   SERVES 4

## FRUITY CAKES   G

100 g (4 oz/1 stick) butter/margarine
100 g (4 oz) unrefined sugar (reduced to
    caster (superfine) sugar consistency in
    a blender or food processor)
2 eggs, beaten

200 g (5½ oz) Trufree No 7 self-raising
    (self-rising) flour, or other wheat-free
    flour
100–150 g (4–6 oz/¾–1 cup) mixed
    raisins, currants and sultanas (golden
    raisins)

Cream butter or margarine and sugar till light and fluffy. Add eggs gradually then fold in flour. Stir in mixed dried fruit. Put mixture into individual cake cases and bake at 190°C (375°F/Mark 5) for 15–18 minutes till risen and golden.

Alternatively place all the mixture in a 500 g (1 lb) loaf tin and cook at 180°C (350°F/Mark 4) for 20–25 minutes for a sweet fruit loaf.   MAKES 10 CAKES

## GINGER BANANAS   G

4 ripe bananas
small amount preserved ginger

25 g (1 oz) flaked almonds

Slice the bananas into individual dishes (one per person). Rinse the syrup from the preserved ginger and chop fairly finely. Sprinkle ginger over the bananas and top with a few almonds.   SERVES 4

**Variation** Mix in a few drops of lemon juice and sprinkle with sunflower seeds.

## EGG CUSTARD   G&Y

175 ml (6 fl oz/¾ cup) milk
2 egg yolks
mild honey to taste

A few drops of real vanilla essence
    (optional)

Heat the milk to boiling point and add slowly to the well-beaten egg yolks. Return to the pan, preferably a double boiler, and stir over a gentle heat until the mixture thickens slightly. Sweeten to taste with honey and add a few drops of vanilla essence if liked. The custard will thicken as it cools.   SERVES 2

# 17

# STRESS OR DISTRESS?

Let's first take a look at the terms stress and distress. In my opinion a certain amount of stress in life gets the adrenaline going and can be both mentally stimulating and healthy. When the pressure rises to the point where it then becomes uncomfortable, you can rest assured that you've hit the band of distress.

Don't ever underestimate the power of distress on your physical and mental well-being. I've seen many a 'strong' person bite the dust when under incredible pressure. The classic case is a person who seems to cope amazingly well with a disaster or a near-tragedy. They sail through the event appearing cool, calm and collected. Then several months later get physically sick or become emotionally unbalanced. It is now understood that stress places extra nutritional demands on the body. And when we are feeling stressed we often don't eat as well as usual, which can make matters worse.

Part of the game is being able to identify the source of stress and admit honestly that you are finding it a strain.

When you are feeling on top of the world physically and mentally your tolerance of problems or particularly difficult situations may be higher. Whereas when you feel below par, extra problems often seem too much to bear.

Many a physical and emotional illness is precipitated by stress. The body's demand for B vitamins increases when under stress. Often, when people have severe problems, their diet suffers and they either eat insufficient food to meet their requirements or indulge in too much junk food and alcohol. You will have seen from Chapter 13 how deficiencies in B vitamins can lead to nervous and mental disorders. Food allergies are also often linked to distressing situations. These can affect the mind and the body. Migraine headaches, irritable bowel syndrome, agoraphobia, diarrhoea, depression, insomnia, nervous tension, mood swings, restlessness, etc. can all result from stress-induced food intolerance.

## A PROBLEM SHARED IS A PROBLEM HALVED

There is no need to pretend you aren't suffering: it's far better to talk over your problems and frustrations, and even have a good cry if you feel like it. Crying can be very therapeutic. Once the problem has been talked through, you may find it gets put a little more into perspective. You may suddenly realize how to cope with the situation immediately, or in the long term. Support and reassurance are very comforting: having a friend to lean on at times of great need is a very valuable asset. There is no substitute for plenty of open, honest communication.

Try to stand outside the problem and examine it clearly. This often helps you to see things more clearly. Sometimes, being so involved in a situation means you can't 'see the wood for the trees'.

Most of all, take time out each day to get your attention off the problem. Consciously daydream, if you like, in a quiet room undisturbed, or go for a long country walk and observe the wonders of nature. Discipline yourself to do this regularly. You'll be surprised how therapeutic these activities can be.

## HOW STRESS AFFECTS YOUR BODY

Pay attention to your body telling you it's not very happy. Look out for possible weak areas that are more susceptible to tension build-up. For example:

| | |
|---|---|
| Forehead | Upper back |
| Face | Lower back |
| Neck | Hands |
| Shoulders | Legs |

Clenched teeth, grinding teeth at night, headaches and eye strain are all signs of inner stress. Becoming aware of your weaknesses is half the battle. The stresses and strains of life do tend to build up in the body. We are each affected differently. Some people suffer backaches, whilst others get headaches. When the body becomes loaded with tension we tie up our energy to some extent. The energy flows become blocked and as a result symptoms like headaches and abdominal cramps are likely to become worse. You can gently massage any tense areas or have someone do it for you, preferably each day. Also try to spend 10–15 minutes at the end of the day consciously relaxing your muscles, beginning with your face and working your way down to your toes.

A good massage is soothing. Yoga may help and it is easy to practise simple relaxing techniques at home. There are other suggestions to help you through difficult periods. Meditation, autogenic training and physical exercise seem to be beneficial for some people. It's really a question of choosing a method of relaxation which you are happy to practise regularly.

There are certain areas in your life which you might like to examine if you are feeling stressed.

- Have you taken on so many commitments that you aren't able to really enjoy life?

  Some people just can't say 'No'. They have good hearts, and little appreciation of their actual working capacity. If you are guilty of this, do sit back and have a good think about it. Make yourself a work schedule and a leisure schedule and stick to it.

- Have you got any goals or aims in life you are pursuing? Having a strong sense of purpose in life is a great asset. Not having a purpose or direction can have repercussions on your mental well-being and subsequently affect your health. Without a desire to achieve something, life often becomes rather boring and meaningless.

- Have you got many unfinished projects on the go, and never seem to get around to finishing any one of them?

  Knowing that you should have completed a project and didn't, especially if it's something promised to another, can be stressful. Make a list of any unfinished projects and then assign a regular time each week, to work through them gradually.

- Is your home and/or work environment tidy and in order, or have you allowed things to pile up around you?

  It is difficult to thrive or relax properly in an area which is untidy, disordered or dirty. If you feel there is room for improvement, why not have a grand 'sort out' or clean up – I'll bet you feel better afterwards.

- Do you have plenty of interests and activities to pursue in your spare time? It is healthy to maintain a wide variety of interests: perhaps some activities that you like to indulge in yourself, and also activities and interests you can share with other members of your family, friends and pets.

- Do you take regular exercise and set aside relaxation time for yourself? Exercise and relaxation are both extremely valuable pursuits and contribute greatly to health. The next chapter is on the subject of exercise and should help you to work out an activity plan.

# 18

# THE VALUE OF EXERCISE AND RELAXATION

I can't emphasize strongly enough how important exercise and relaxation are in maintaining a healthy body. There have been several studies which demonstrated that exercise was a valuable tool in overcoming depression, and the PMT A symptoms of nervous tension, mood swings, irritability and anxiety.

If you don't like structural exercises you should at least take a brisk walk for half an hour a day. Personally I find swimming one of the most stimulating exercises, especially at the start of the day.

Beyond doubt, exercise raises energy levels, and your spirits. On a regular basis, it also speeds up the metabolism of the body. Although you may have to push yourself initially, I assure you it will pay dividends within a short space of time.

The mind and body work closely together. The mental stress of PMT will be reflected in the physical tension in your body. The muscular aches and pains of PMT such as headaches, neck pain and stiff joints, together with the more obvious low backache and abdominal cramps, all work to increase feelings of anxiety and depression. It's hardly surprising that the heart rate increases, as the nervous and physical tension increases, all adding to feelings of being 'wound up'.

Exercise may provide help for PMT sufferers more than just by acting as a general tonic. Recently, it has been shown that the level of a particular brain hormone, beta-endorphin, a hormone associated with a sense of well-being and pain relief, was found to be low in pre-menstrual sufferers in the few days before their period. The levels during the first phase of the menstrual cycle were normal when compared with healthy women who did not have PMT. Beta-endorphin is an important self-produced hormone, which may affect mood and well-being, and also influence the function of other hormones. Its level can be raised by regular and usually prolonged physical exercise. Potentially, it could also be influenced by dietary and nutritional factors.

Thus, regular physical exercise by stimulating the body's natural production of beta-endorphin might help to prevent the dip that occurs pre-menstrually in PMT sufferers. Other studies have shown that physical exercise can be of value in the treatment of depression.

## GENERAL ADVICE

- It is important to take time off to care for yourself.

- Ensure that exercise and relaxation become part of your daily lifestyle.

- Choose styles of exercise that suit your personality and lifestyle.

- Make an effort to slow down at the critical time and look to ways of calming your mind and body – particularly important if your coordination suffers and you become clumsy.

- Above all, take a programme of exercise that balances the 3 'S's with some 'R' – universally known as:

### STRENGTH, STAMINA, SUPPLENESS AND RELAXATION

Taking each of the elements in turn, I have highlighted the important factors.

**S for Strength** can be described as the maximum force needed by a muscle or group of muscles to overcome a resistance.

In everyday terms this means being able to push, pull, lift, climb and carry without injuring yourself. Strong back and abdominal muscles will help improve your posture and guard you from most lower back pain.

There is another important element of strength to consider and that is:

**E for Endurance** is the muscle's ability repeatedly to perform or maintain a task for a prolonged period of time.

There is also cardiovascular (heart and blood vessel function) training which partners muscular endurance training. Different forms of activity will improve the endurance qualities of different muscle groups. For example, running will train the leg muscles much more than the upper body and arms, while swimming will emphasize upper body endurance. Both, however, will increase cardiovascular endurance.

**S for Stamina** simply means being able to keep going; whether you're walking, swimming, running or cycling – and without stopping or becoming tired!

These types of activity are called 'aerobic' because of the increased need for oxygen by the working muscles. Remember, the heart is a muscle too and it needs exercise just as much as your legs or arms. The lungs are used to oxygenate the blood. With regular exercise, the heart and lungs become more efficient. The benefits of aerobic training mean you eventually achieve better results with less effort. Your heart and lungs will have to work less hard in daily life.

Experts disagree as to exactly how much aerobic exercise you need to benefit or gain from the training effect. It will also vary from person to person. A general rule of thumb is to aim for at least 20 minutes about three times a week.

**S for Suppleness** and flexibility: the ability to move your joints through their full range of movement. In other words, being able to bend, stretch, reach and turn to your fullest. Of all the fitness elements so far, flexibility must rate as the one most likely to affect your everyday life. It also means protecting your muscles and joints from injury and stiffness, as well as improving your circulation, posture and poise.

Improving your range of movement will also help to improve your performance in other activities. Correct stretching, when practised after your exercise session (as well as before), will help to minimize the likelihood of post-exercise soreness.

**R for Relaxation** is the art of letting go. Knowing how to let go and with confidence, is probably one of the most important elements of health and fitness. The ability to release unnecessary muscular tension and calm the mind is a wonderful resource to call upon. Tension is tiring and unproductive.

For some, exercise itself is a form of relaxation, while others might turn to a hobby or pastime.

Relaxation and breathing go hand in hand. Indeed, improving your breathing patterns during exercise is one of the keys to success. It also engenders a feeling of alertness and readiness to cope.

Over the weeks of a considered programme of exercise you will increase the efficiency of your heart and lung capacity with deeper breathing.

## TIPS AND HINTS ON EXERCISING

To really ensure you gain the maximum benefit from your efforts, take a few moments to read the following tips and hints – they make all the difference to how you feel about your exercising.

- Remember, exercise should be fun and something you look forward to.
- It won't be if you push yourself fast and furiously, it will only leave you exhausted, sore and disappointed with your efforts.
- Really listen to your body. Believe it or not, it knows best!
- Take it slowly and gradually for longer-lasting results.
- Take time to work out your fitness aims and objectives – what do you want to achieve from your efforts? Finding and following the right programme for you is as vital as eating the right food.
- Decide which activity, or blend of activites, will suit you and help to realize your aims.
- Mix and match whenever possible. Avoid boredom by choosing from several activities you know that you will enjoy and stick at. Better still, are they convenient and can you enjoy the company of others at the same time?
- Try to combine some of your exercises with fresh air and sunlight, both of which have proven benefit in helping to relieve PMT symptoms.
- Balance is the key to successful exercising. Give upper and lower body the same amount of work and spread the load.
- Don't expect miracles overnight – be patient and persevere!
- Aim for quality of exercise, not quantity – look forward to it and enjoy it.

## PRECAUTIONS

Most people do not need a full medical check-up before exercising, but if you answer YES to any of the following questions, or you are over 35 and a 'first timer', it's best to discuss your plans with your doctor.

Have you ever suffered from, or is there a family history of:

Chest pains or pain in the shoulders?
High blood pressure or heart disease?
Chest problems like asthma or bronchitis?
Back pain or joint pains?
Headaches, faintness or feelings of nausea?
Diabetes?
Are you taking any medication?
Are you recovering from illness or recent operations?
Are you very overweight?
Are you pregnant?

If you have a cold or sore throat, give exercise a miss until you feel better. When you do resume, take it slowly and build up to your pre-illness fitness level gradually. If you ever feel pain, dizziness, nausea or undue tiredness whenever or wherever you exercise, STOP immediately. Rest and wait. Change your position or slacken off the intensity if relevant. Try again. If the complaint persists, stop and seek professional advice.

### Posture pointers

- Stand in front of a full-length mirror with feet about hip-width apart and insteps lifted.

- Gently rock back and forth to find your balance and 'centred' position. Body-weight will feel evenly balanced between balls and heels, as well as inner and outer edges of feet.

- Line knees directly over ankles and gently pull up thigh muscles above the knees.

### The standing position

Now stand sideways to the mirror. Push your bottom out and see and feel the lower back arch and tummy bulge. Correct this by pulling in the abdominal muscles and tucking the buttocks under you. See and feel the lower back lengthen as the pubic bone (pelvis) tilts up to the ceiling. This is the pelvic tilt.

- Keep hips level and maintain pelvic tilt as you turn to face mirror.

- Lift ribcage up and away from hips.

- Pull shoulders down from ears; keep them level and aligned over ankles.

- Let arms hang loosely.

- Lift head upwards from crown and feel the back of neck lengthen.

- Hold chin at right angle to ground.

- Feel entire spine lengthen.

Run through these posture pointers and the pelvic tilt frequently throughout the day, to maintain alignment and heighten your awareness.

### Warm up

Now you're ready to warm up. Never miss out this section as it prepares your body for the work to follow. Mobilizing and loosening exercises, plus some preliminary

202

stretches, will help to improve your performance and skill by increasing the body temperature. A warm up also helps to reduce the risk of injury and soreness. About 10 minutes is all most people need. Similarly, 'warm down' at the end of each session – no matter how rushed you are. End with some rhythmical exercises and slow holding stretches that taper down from more demanding ones. A warm-down will induce a feeling of relaxation and well-being. It will also help to reduce the likelihood of post-exercise stiffness and soreness.

Warm up by moving rhythmically for ten minutes to your favourite piece of music, working from your feet upwards, gradually using your whole body.

During your warm-down, take it easy, hold your stretches and slow down gradually. This will minimize any soreness and stiffness.

### Relieve the tension

This section takes a look at specific exercises and steps you can take to release tension associated with PMT, as well as improve posture and awareness.

Deeper breathing will be promoted, as well as relaxation and a feeling of calm.

### Shoulders and neck

Tension and tightness generally collect at the base of the neck and across tops of shoulders. They are mostly due to the way we sit and stand, as well as being our natural reaction to stress – we slouch, so the neck collapses and the shoulders hunch. Not a pretty sight and often it leaves us with a headache due to the constriction of blood supply to and from the brain.

Take positive steps to overcome these problems by loosening shoulders and paying more attention to posture. See posture pointers on page 202.

To start, stand or sit well with the head centred and breathe well as you:

1.   Lift both shoulders up, pull them back and strongly down. Repeat several times.

     **Tip – Make sure you really squeeze into the upper back and keep chin held in.**

2.   Clasp hands loosely behind lower back and rest them just above buttocks.

     Keep elbows bent and hand resting on body throughout.

     Squeeze between the shoulder blades so the elbows draw together.

     Hold and release slowly.

     Repeat several times.

Feel the squeeze between the shoulder blades and the stretch across the chest.

**Tip – Keep the shoulders down, head centred and lower back straight.**

3. Turn head slowly to look over right shoulder while maintaining length in the neck and keeping shoulders still.

   Return to centre and repeat to opposite side.

   Repeat several times.

   Return to centre and pull chin in to lengthen back of neck.

   Tilt head slowly to right shoulder while keeping shoulders level.

   Feel the stretch on the opposite side.

   Return slowly to centre.

   **Tip – As you tilt head, imagine you are looking into a mirror to see both cheeks evenly.**

   Finally, return to centre, pull shoulders down and tuck chin in.

   Tilt head gently forwards.

   Feel the stretch along the neck.

   Return to centre and repeat once more, breathing well.

### Back and hips

1. **Back strengthener**

   Lie on your front on either a mat or rug, with legs together, forehead on floor and chin tucked in.

   Clasp hands loosely and rest them on lower back.

   As you breathe out, contract abdominal and buttock muscles and squeeze between the shoulder blades.

   Straighten arms down towards your feet and raise chest, shoulders and forehead off the floor to form one continuous line.

   Lower slowly to the floor and repeat once more.

204

## 2.  Back release

From the previous exercise, place hands under shoulders and gently push up onto your knees to lower your bottom back onto your heels.

Fold your body forwards to rest chest on thighs.

Tuck your head down and rest arms down by sides of body.

**Tip – If you feel claustrophobic, stretch your arms out in front of you and rest forehead lightly on floor.**

## 3.  Pelvic tilt

Use the pelvic tilt as a back release as well as a preliminary movement to abdominal strengtheners.

Pelvic tilts can be done standing, sitting or lying. Take time to practise the movement, as getting it right makes all the difference to the safety and effectiveness of your exercising and alignment.

Start by lying back on a mat or rug.

Bend knees with feet hip-width apart and lengthen back of neck by tucking chin in.

As you breathe out, press lower back down on to mat and pull in abdominal muscles.

Feel the pubic bone tilt up to the ceiling and the lower back flatten down against the floor.

Practise several times until you feel confident of the movement.

## 4.  Curl-overs to strengthen abdominal muscles

Strong abdominal muscles help prevent some lower back pain.

Start as for the pelvic tilt and rest hands on your thighs.

As you breathe out, pelvic tilt and curl head and shoulders slowly off the floor, sliding hands toward knees.

Hold for count of four with waist and lower back on floor.

Lie back slowly and repeat four times.

### Let go!

Having the ability to release tension and calm the mind is a wonderful resource to call upon. Tension is tiring and wasteful. Knowing how to cope and apply positive resources is the key to successful relaxation. Adopt any position you find comfortable and supportive for your lower back and neck. It may mean sitting in a high-back chair, or lying back with neck supported by a cushion and legs resting on a chair or stool.

Use your breathing to enhance your relaxation and let your restorative side take over.

Remember to pull the shoulders well down from the ears and let arms rest heavily.

Take several deep breaths, feeling the ribcage move up and out like bellows as you breathe in, and downwards as you breathe out.

Your breathing will gradually become more rhythmical as you start to let go.

Run down your body and check where you feel tight.

Are your shoulders up round your ears? Pull them down. Are your hands clenched? Stretch them out and let the fingers curl.

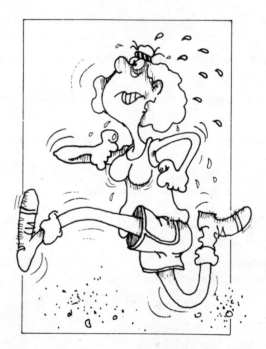

What about your buttocks and lower back? Make an extra effort to relax and release – try the pelvic tilt to prevent back arching.

Concentrate on your legs, particularly ankles and feet. Let them go and feel the whole body soften.

Finally pay attention to your mouth and face. Soften the jaw and let the softness spread over your face – around the nostrils, between and over your eyes and across your forehead to your hairline.

Spend a few quiet moments with yourself.

When you feel ready, take a few deep breaths, have a good stretch and yawn before curling over to one side and sitting up slowly.

# 19

# OTHER VALUABLE
# THERAPIES

As well as dealing with symptoms on a nutritional level it is important to make sure that your whole body is functioning at optimum level. The years during which you may have suffered nutritional deficiencies, while coping with stressful situations and pre-menstrual symptoms, may well have taken their toll on your body. The body is a very complicated, but delicate network of bones, muscles, ligaments, nerves, organs and blood vessels. Physical symptoms and nervous tension can affect the smooth running of the body processes. When you make a start on your nutritional programme, if your symptoms are intense, you might consider the value of osteopathy, cranial osteopathy, acupuncture, or acupressure. They are powerful tools and can help to bring about speedy relief of symptoms.

## OSTEOPATHY

It is not uncommon, through the wear and tear of everyday life, for subtle back or neck problems to occur. I have seen many resistant, long-standing headaches cured by some good osteopathic manipulation. It is certainly worth having a check-up with a qualified osteopath if you feel tension building up in your back or neck, or if you suffer regular headaches.

Cranial osteopathy, or cranio-sacral therapy as it is known, is a specialized form of osteopathy. Unlike conventional osteopathy, it is a gentle yet potent form of therapy. The aim is gently to coax the muscles, tendons, joints and connective tissue to establish correct functions and release restrictions, thus restoring normal circulation, flow of energy and glandular secretions.

The cranio-sacral mechanism is comprised of the cranium (the skull), the sacrum (the bone at the base of the spine), the membranes surrounding the brain, the spinal cord and the fascia of continuous, clingfilm-like sheet that surrounds the muscles, organs, joints and bones. The tension of this fascia, the clingfilm-like lining, is all important. If you have ever worn an all-in-one pants suit that is too tight or too short in the body, you will have experienced some discomfort. If the tension in the body's fascia becomes too tight, you can't just take it off like an uncomfortable piece of clothing, and it is possible that body functions can be affected in the long term.

Cranial osteopaths claim a good success rate with women who have PMT and other menstrual disorders. You will find it very gentle treatment. Here are some experiences of a cranial osteopath who regularly treats women with PMT and menstrual problems. As well as her treatment she recommends that her patients take regular exercise and seek nutritional advice.

### Case history 1

The patient experienced migraine and PMT for five to six days prior to each period. She had some lower back strain, reduced mobility in her upper neck and some pelvic congestion. Her neck was treated and normal function restored. As a result, the congestion and strain within the skull were reduced, the migraines were instantly alleviated, and the PMT symptoms reduced. The patient then received nutritional advice and her PMT reduced further.

### Case history 2

This patient was a woman aged 44 who suffered with severe PMT, and backache before and during her period. She was very tall and had poor posture. When examined, she had restricted movement in the lower back and pelvic congestion. After treatment over a period of two months she became 90 per cent better.

It is certainly worth finding a local practitioner if you feel the need is there. (See page 228.)

## ACUPUNCTURE AND ACUPRESSURE

It is worth mentioning the contribution made by traditional Chinese medicine in the treatment of female health problems. According to the severity of the problem, there are two levels at which treatment can be taken. The first level is appropriate for severe symptoms and involves consulting an acupuncturist. Many of the problems mentioned, including PMT, painful periods, irregular periods, fluid retention and distension, pelvic inflammation, migraines, backache, morning sickness and other troubles of pregnancy, menopausal symptoms, depression, anxiety and insomnia may all respond to treatment by acupuncture. If you feel your complaint is too serious or persistent to cope with by yourself, acupuncture is worth considering as a possible option.

Of course you should always ensure that you get help from a properly trained and registered practitioner. You can usually obtain information from your public library or Citizens Advice Bureau. A register is published by the Council for Acupuncture, listing all members of the four recognized and affiliated professional bodies.

As we are concentrating on aspects of self-help, it is worth considering a second level of treatment, more appropriate to the minor or occasional problems which you can sometimes alleviate by self-assessment and treatment at home. This can be done through Shiatsu, the Japanese finger pressure method (sometimes called acupressure). In this system the body is influenced in various ways by stimulating key points, found along the course of energy channels circulating near the skin surface. These are the same as acupuncture meridians, but the points are stimulated by pressure rather than needles.

For Shiatsu to be effective it is important to give the right kind of pressure, for an appropriate length of time. It is no good pushing pressure points like 'magic buttons' and it is important to recognize by the feel whether what you are doing is correct. Provided you adopt the right approach, Shiatsu may be very helpful, whether you enlist the help of a friend or perform it on your own (self-Shiatsu).

Here is a summary of the method and a description of how to find just a few of the most useful points for some of the troubles mentioned.

### Pre-menstrual depression/anxiety

First, try working along the inner leg. Also, two inches above the wrist, in between the tendons at the centre of the inner arm, there is a good point to press firmly. Breathing is very important to get your energy flowing smoothly, so try this simple exercise. Kneel on a cushion or carpeted floor and join your hands together with the fingers back to back while pointing the fingertips towards your own upper abdomen. Let your relaxed fingers press into the centre, below the ribs but above the navel. As you do this lean gently forward and exhale. The pressure should lend a little force to the exhalation. Wait for the inhalation to come naturally and raise yourself back again to the upright kneeling position while breathing in. Go gently at first, repeating the action with every breath, leaning a bit further onto your fingers each time. The abdominal muscles may seem tight or tender but try to relax fully at the end of each breath while leaning forward. Only do this ten times. You may move your fingers up and down or a little way along the ribs to explore for any tension. Afterwards sit quietly for a minute. You may feel like a good stretch before getting up.

## Insomnia/headaches

Work with your own fingertips along the base of the skull behind the head where it joins the neck. Feel for any sensitive hollows where the muscles meet the bony ridge and, leaning your head back, let your fingers penetrate and hold for a few breaths. (If you do this for a friend, support her forehead with one hand and use your other hand to find points with finger and thumb on either side of her neck, pressing inward and upward.) For frontal headaches lean forward, letting your fingertips support the forehead just below the eyebrows – it may feel tender, but breathe and relax for several seconds. Also, work generally along the inside edges and soles of the feet, pressing especially around the inside ankle area. Another useful point for headaches can be found by pressing hard into the fleshy area between your finger and thumb – press towards the edge of the bone on the forefinger side.

## Period pains

Get comfortable. Feel for sensitive points along the inside of the lower leg between the edge of the bone and the calf muscle. Hold any points with sustained thumb-pressure to the limit of comfort for five or six seconds or longer. You should try to breathe easily in a relaxed way and maintain the pressure until the sensation diminishes a little. To make it easier, reinforce one thumb with the other while pressing. Ask a friend or partner to lean with their thumbs into the area of the sacrum (triangular bony part at the base of your spine between the buttocks), they could explore a little way each side of centre, pressing firmly but gently any tender spots they find (you should say if it is too strong).

If this approach really interests you, there are two particularly good books you could read which are mentioned on the Reading List on page 226. You could also look for Shiatsu classes in your area. If you do not know of any, write to the secretary of the Shiatsu Society whose address is listed in Appendix 6 at the back of the book, page 229. The Society will send you a list of qualified teachers.

Whatever you do, it is important to ensure that you put yourself in the hands of a qualified practitioner. These days all the recognized alternative therapies have official associations. These bodies keep registers of qualified practitioners. It is best to check up as there are, sadly, quite a few non-qualified practitioners who are not to be recommended.

# 20

# OTHER NUTRITIONALLY RELATED PROBLEMS

If you have identified your PMT symptoms and carefully followed the nutritional programme, yet you still experience troublesome symptoms, it may be that there is some other hindrance at work.

In this chapter I will look at several 'stumbling blocks' which also have to be taken into account. You may need to make changes in your nutritional programme in the light of one of these specific problems.

## MENOPAUSE

It is an accepted fact that as women get older, their PMT symptoms get worse, if untreated. The menopause usually occurs during the late forties and early fifties, although it can begin earlier.

The most common menopausal symptoms seem to be as follows:

| | |
|---|---|
| Hot flushes | Headaches |
| Dizziness | Depression |
| Lethargy | Insomnia |
| Nervousness | Decreased sex drive |
| Poor memory | Dry vagina |

Hormone Replacement Therapy (HRT) is often suggested but is not really desirable in the long term. Most women seem to prefer a more natural approach rather than taking hormones for years on end.

Once again moderate sufferers could follow Option 2 of the PMT programme. It is likely that the more severe sufferers have nutritional deficiencies and respond well to a personal nutritional programme. This would include specific dietary changes and supplements recommended according to the symptoms present, and other related factors. If the problem can be handled by nutritional means, it seems to make far more sense to tackle it in this way rather than continuing to take artificial substances.

You are better off seeking professional advice than going on suffering indefinitely. Once again, you will find that the Women's Nutritional Advisory Service is equipped to help menopausal sufferers over their symptoms, address on page 228.

## POST-NATAL DEPRESSION

Many women develop severe PMT symptoms after having children, when they have not suffered before.

Post-natal depression can be very severe when it strikes and can last for many months, and in extreme cases, even longer. To my knowledge no good studies have been done to look at the correlation between post-natal depression and nutritional state. We have, over the years, been able to help many post-natal depression sufferers by providing a diet and supplement programme, in the same way we would for PMT or menopause sufferers.

One particular patient had had severe post-natal depression after the births of both of her children. She also developed PMT severely. We were able to clear up her PMT completely by helping her through a nutritional programme. She then followed our maintenance plan and continued with a good diet and reduced her dosage of supplements. A year later she became pregnant again, and followed some nutritional suggestions we made for her pregnancy. Her third baby was born and she felt well. She has not experienced any post-natal depression whatsoever. Compared to when we first met up, she is now in far better nutritional shape, which I feel sure was the key to her problem.

## PERIOD PAIN

Period pains are particularly common in teenagers and women in their early twenties. Characteristically, as they disappear, so pre-menstrual symptoms tend to appear and get worse. There are many cases of painful periods and some of these will only respond to medical treatment. If you have persistently painful periods you should be checked by your own doctor. But many girls know that their periods are just painful for one or two days, particularly if they pass clots at the start of their

213

period. Large quantities of aspirin and other painkillers are now sold to young women because of period pains, but other treatments may be more helpful.

One study has shown that 50 mg of vitamin E, three times per day can be helpful with period pains. Bioflavonoids, a type of compound related to vitamin C and found in high concentrations in citrus fruits and yellow and green vegetables, have been shown to help some women with painful periods. Doses of about 500 mg per day before the period and four days after it starts have resulted in an improvement in three-quarters of the young women in one study.

It is possible, too, that by changing the diet, periods can become less painful: cutting down on animal fats and ensuring a good intake of magnesium, B vitamins and vitamin C may be beneficial. Losing weight, if overweight, and taking physical exercise should also help.

## HEAVY AND IRREGULAR PERIODS

Heavy and irregular periods can affect women at any time in their childbearing years. Being overweight can be a significant cause because of its effect on the hormone metabolism, thus it may be important to lose weight. Heavy periods can lead to iron deficiency, anaemia, which can in fact aggravate the period problems; hence the correction of any iron deficiency or anaemia is essential.

Sometimes just improving one's diet may be of benefit to heavy and irregular periods. Certainly, if there is an excess consumption of alcohol, this should be modified. Any women with persistently heavy or irregular periods or abnormal bleeding should consult their medical practitioner.

## STERILIZATION

It seems that after sterilization or other gynaecological procedures, symptoms can suddenly occur with a vengeance. This in fact happened to Jane, who you read about in Part One.

> 'Ever since I was sterilized I had PMT symptoms. I never had any kind of PMT or period problems before. I went back to the doctor who sterilized me when I started to get these symptoms every month. He just turned around and said, "You women are all the same. You don't want any more babies, we sterilize you and then you come back and complain."

> The doctor assured me that sterilization had nothing to do with the symptoms I was getting now, but I insisted that before the sterilization I had felt perfectly OK, terrific every month and did not have any PMT symptoms whatsoever. I was very annoyed by his reaction.'

214

Why symptoms suddenly arrive is not really understood, although it is believed progesterone levels drop for a while after sterilization. However, we have managed to eliminate the symptoms once again with the nutritional programme. Obviously, much more research is needed into the whole issue of the implications of nutritional deficiencies.

# 21

# MEN WHO NO
# LONGER SUFFER

I didn't feel that the book would be complete without giving a voice to the men in our lives. I have concentrated so far on how women suffer with PMT. But it's not just women who suffer, let's face it, the men are very definitely on the receiving end! Women who have supportive partners have a far easier time on the programme than those whose partners refuse to acknowledge the condition and instead of being understanding, just simply fight back and turn off.

I have had the good fortune to hear from many men who were deeply concerned about the welfare of their women, once they understood that PMT was a real condition, which would respond to treatment.

I think it's important for women to stand back and examine some of the viewpoints, in retrospect, of men who have lived with PMT sufferers before, during and after their nutritional programme. I'm happy to say they can mostly look back and laugh, probably with relief, for the storm is over.

Tom Moor, Jane's husband, is relieved to say that he got back the girl he married.

> 'Jane was very irritable, she couldn't hold a conversation without snapping. I couldn't touch her for two weeks before her periods as her breasts were so sore and tender. She rarely wanted to go out and would make excuses to stay at home. When she had PMT she changed from being very happy-go-lucky to being bitchy, irritable and tired.

> When she was pre-menstrual I used to keep out of her way. I still showed her that I loved her and waited patiently for her one good week each month. We were hoping for an early menopause.

> The nutritional programme has made a tremendous difference to our lives. We are able to lead a normal life again. My wife laughs and jokes and she is popular at work.

*My advice to other men is to seek help as it is available. Once their partner is on a nutritional programme, help her to persevere, as it will pay dividends in the long run. I feel that more education for men is necessary, more widespread information directed at couples. I, like most men, was totally baffled as to what the cause of the problem was.'*

Don, June Garson's husband couldn't imagine what the consequences might have been had she not received help.

*'Generally speaking I am a calm, tolerant person. I tried to make allowances, but I didn't understand the problem. It was like living with a "time bomb" not knowing when it was going to go off! June was permanently "uptight" and tearful pre-menstrually. She was unable to cope with life or deal with the children rationally.*

*Once on the nutritional programme an immediate improvement was noticeable. Her new-found state of mind and feeling of well-being turned the clock back to the time when we met, prior to our children being born. She reverted back personality-wise to the girl I fell for. I no longer dread the time of the month.*

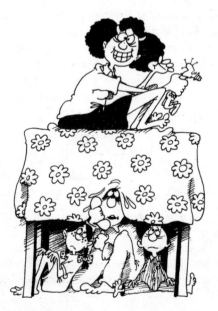

*My advice to other men is as follows:*

*Be totally committed to discussing the subject in detail with your partner, read extensively on the subject and INSIST on her seeking help, not only for her sake, but for the rest of the family. Ignorance of the subject is the major hurdle to overcome.*

*I found your literature and your "cure" very interesting as I employ 150 people, many of them women. As a result of my experience with my wife I was able to realize that a staff problem affecting many employees was due to the PMT of a particular female employee. I have been able to discuss her problem sympathetically and we hope to solve the unrest in the office, as on my recommendation she has written to you for your help.'*

Nadine's boyfriend felt that the biggest change for him was that he no longer had to duck to avoid the flying saucepans!

*'Nadine's hysterical and often violent acts of throwing objects did cause anger, but more usefully, it improved my reaction time and my catching abilities no end!'*

Life was difficult to cope with for Nadine. There were times of great frustration when new remedies for PMT failed to work. Since introducing the nutritional programme into her life, the quality of life for Nadine and her partner has increased enormously.

*'I think the key to coping with PMT is to be patient and caring. If her irritability makes you irritable, then feel it, but don't show it. If her hysteria is frightening then allow yourself to be afraid, but be bigger than your fear, and calm her down. Be practical, do the cooking or take over the task she is finding difficult to cope with. Give up your time because you can bet she's feeling worse than you've ever done, and deserves your understanding and a shoulder to lean on. Tell her you love her and reassure her, and most of all, mean it.'*

This bittersweet excerpt is from a letter written by the husband of one of our patients:

*'I am Dodd, a roofing contractor with eight children and a wife with severe PMT symptoms. She was a complete Jekyll and Hyde character when her PMT struck.*

*Knowing what divorce can do to a family, I had to have the patience of Job with Eleanor. But after violent attacks (both on myself and the children), outrageous outbursts, locking herself into hotel rooms, insults, screams of rage, alienation from reality, a suicide attempt, and jealous behaviour I had had it. Bearing in mind that for most of the month she was warm, affectionate and everything a wife should be.*

*The worst of it all was after an attack when the illness had left her and she would creep back to me. Then I had to play the part of the caring husband again.*

*How can you expect a young couple with two children to come to terms with this terrible PMT problem when there is nowhere to go, nobody to see them? PMT is a dreadful affliction. It is self-destructive, life-threatening and family-life threatening. When I was a child, I would go to see a horror film and on it would be a pit of snakes – provided you did not disturb them they left you alone but woe betide you if you disturbed them. It was the same with Eleanor if she stuck to the diet or went on a binge.*

*Women are such beautiful creatures, advanced both mentally and physically from the male. More adaptable, stronger, philosophical, and yet they have to cope with some of the most awful female problems. Is this the price a woman has to pay for her beauty?*

*Eleanor is now cured of her PMT symptoms. I know she is cured and the WNAS has been responsible. The reason (after trying everything else) I know they have hit the nail on the head is because if complacency sets in and she starts pinching sweets, eating curries and drinking, I can guarantee by the end of her monthly cycle she will be going through agony. I am eternally grateful.'*

His advice to other men is as follows:

1. *A woman has to realize that she has a problem and that it is not everybody else around her that is wrong, but herself.*

2. *If and when she realizes this, she is 49% there.*

3. *She has to get the husband to realize (buy him a dummy to suck; he will need it to bite hard on). You are then 98% there.*

4. *The last 2% is really just the beginning. When it has been realized, you still have an awful long way to go. But it is like everything else in life, you do not get owt for nowt. This now is when you really have to work hard. It is just like any other illness – if left untreated, it just gets worse.*

Isn't that great? What wonderful understanding! The common factor for most men who are supportive, seems to be that they were educated on the subject of PMT. When they don't understand what's going on, they obviously find it more difficult to be supportive in the long term, which is quite understandable.

On behalf of PMT sufferers I would like to thank the supportive men of the world for being willing to share the problem. With more education, communication and understanding in the future on the subject of PMT, far fewer lives will be needlessly disrupted.

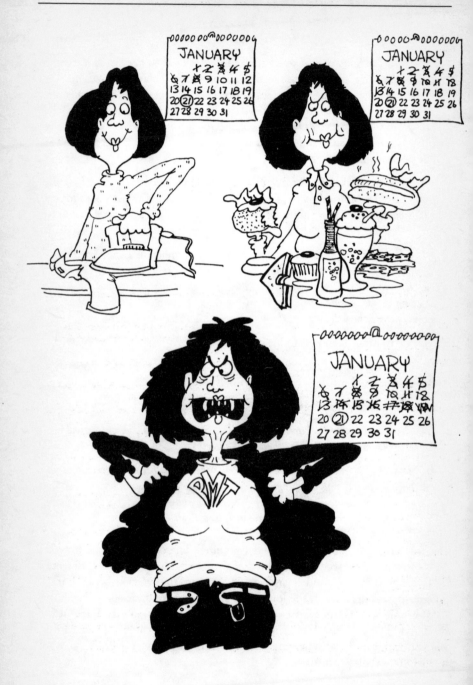

# 1  DICTIONARY OF TERMS

**Abbreviations used**

g = gram, mg = milligram (100 mg = 1 g), mcg = microgram (100 mcg = 1 mg), iu = international unit, kj = kilojoule

**ADRENAL GLANDS.** The adrenal glands are two small glands situated at the top of the kidneys. They produce several different hormones, most of which are steroid hormones. Hormones from the adrenal glands influence the metabolism of sugar, salt and water and several other functions.

**ALDACTONE.** This is a diuretic drug which helps fluid retention. It inhibits the action of aldosterone, a hormone from the adrenal glands. It is also known as spironolactone.

**ALDOSTERONE.** This is a steroid hormone produced by the adrenal glands which is involved in salt and water balance. When it is produced in excess it causes the body to hold water and sodium salt.

**ALLERGY.** An unusual and unexpected sensitivity to a particular substance which causes an adverse reaction. Foods, chemicals and environmental pollutants are common irritants and they may cause a whole range of symptoms including headaches, abdominal bloating and discomfort, skin rashes, eczema and asthma.

**AMENORRHOEA.** A complete absence of periods.

**AMINO ACIDS.** Chains of building blocks which combine together to form the proteins that make living things. There are some 20 or more amino acids, some of which are essential and some non-essential.

**ANTI-DEPRESSANTS.** These are drugs used to suppress symptoms of depression.

**BROMOCRIPTINE.** A powerful drug, used to suppress the hormone prolactin. Further details of this can be found in Chapter 12, on conventional remedies. It is occasionally used in the treatment of PMT.

**CARBOHYDRATES.** Carbohydrates are the main source of calories (kjs) in almost all diets.
*Complex carbohydrates* are essential nutrients and occur in the form of fruits, vegetables, pulses and grains. They are important energy-giving foods. There are two sorts of complex carbohydrates: the first are digestible, such as the starches, and the second are not digestible and are more commonly known as 'fibre'.
*Refined carbohydrates.* These consist of foods that have been processed and refined. White or brown sugar and white flour have, in the process of refining, had many of the vitamins and minerals present in the original plant removed. Further details on this may be found in Chapter 11.

**CERVIX.** The neck of the womb which projects downwards into the vagina.

**CORPUS LUTEUM.** Literally, a little yellow gland or body. It is the part of the ovary that remains after the egg has left. It produces two hormones, oestrogen and progesterone, during the second half of the menstrual cycle.

**DAY 1 OF CYCLE.** The first day of the menstrual bleeding, the day the period arrives, is the first day of the menstrual cycle.

**DEFICIENCY.** A lack of an essential substance, e.g. a vitamin.

**DIURETICS.** Drugs which cause an increased production of urine by the kidneys. They are used to treat fluid retention.

**DOPAMINE.** Dopamine is a brain chemical affecting mood. It has a sedating effect.

**DYSMENORRHOEA.** This is a term used to describe pain occurring during periods.

**ENDOCRINE GLANDS.** Glands that secrete hormones and regulate other organs in the body. The thyroid and the pituitary glands are endocrine glands.

**ENDOMETRIOSIS.** A condition in which the lining of the uterus begins to grow outside the uterus in the abdominal cavity. It is usually a painful condition and can be a cause of infertility.

**ENDORPHINS.** Hormones from the pituitary gland and fluid in the spine which are believed to help control moods, behaviour and part of the workings of the pituitary gland itself. They may also have an effect on how sugar is used in the body, and on other amounts of hormones released from the pituitary gland and the ovaries. If this is so, the production of oestrogen and progesterone could be affected by endorphins.

**ESSENTIAL FATTY ACIDS.** One of the essential groups of foods which we need to eat to remain healthy. These are essential fats that are necessary for normal cell structure and body function. There are two: linoleic and linolenic acids. They are called 'essential' as they cannot be made by the body but have to be eaten in the diet.

**FALLOPIAN TUBES.** A pair of slender tubes through which the egg passes on its way from the ovary to the uterus. Fertilization occurs in the Fallopian tubes. Very rarely the egg remains in the tube and grows: this is called an ectopic pregnancy, and is a medical emergency accompanied by severe abdominal pain.

**FOLLICLE.** A small sac in the ovary containing an egg (ovum). After release of the egg at mid cycle the follicle becomes a corpus luteum.

**FOLLICLE STIMULATING HORMONE (FSH).** A hormone of the pituitary gland which stimulates the growth of the follicles in the ovaries.

**FOLLICULAR PHASE.** The first half of the menstrual cycle when an egg is growing in the ovary. The egg is surrounded by cells which produce the hormone oestrogen and which thus prepares the uterus for conception. The egg and surrounding cells are called a follicle.

**GLUCOSE.** A form of sugar, found in the diet or released by the liver into the bloodstream, which is then used by the brain for energy. This is the only source of energy usable by the brain.

**GRAAFIAN FOLLICLE.** A mature egg which is surrounded by a bag of fluid within the ovary.

**HORMONES.** Substances formed chiefly in the endocrine glands, which then enter the bloodstream and control the activity of an organ or body function. Adrenaline and insulin are hormones, as are oestrogen and progesterone.

**HYPERHYDRATION – too much water present.** This is a term used to describe water retention in the body.

**HYPOGLYCAEMIA – LOW BLOOD SUGAR.** This is a condition in which there is a deficiency of glucose in the bloodstream, often caused by an excess of insulin or a lack of food. As glucose is required for normal brain function, mental disturbance can occur as can other symptoms: headaches, weakness, faintness, irritability, palpitations, mood swings, sweating and hunger. One of the commonest contributing factors is an excess of refined carbohydrates in the diet.

**HYPOTHALAMUS.** The region of the brain controlling temperature, hunger, thirst and the hormones produced by the pituitary gland.

**HYSTERECTOMY.** A surgical procedure to remove the womb and the Fallopian tubes. Sometimes one or more ovaries are also removed.

**LUTEAL PHASE.** The time after the egg has left the follicle in the ovary, and the follicle then becomes a gland known as the corpus luteum. The corpus luteum produces progesterone.

**LUTEINIZING HORMONE (LH).** The pituitary hormone which fosters the development of the corpus luteum.

**MENORRHAGIA.** An excessive loss of blood during each period.

**MENSES.** The discharge of blood and tissue lining from the uterus, which occurs approximately every four weeks between puberty and the menopause.

**MENSTRUAL CYCLE.** The monthly cycle involving the pituitary gland, ovaries and uterus in which an egg is produced ready for conception to take place. In each cycle an egg in the ovary is released and the lining of the womb develops ready for conception and implantation of the fertilized egg. If this does not occur, the lining of the womb is shed and a period occurs.

**MENSTRUAL SYMPTOMATOLOGY DIARY.** A chart which is a daily record of all symptoms that occur throughout the menstrual cycle.

**METABOLISM.** The process by which the body maintains life. It is the cycle of nutrients being broken down to produce energy, which is then used by the body to build up new cells and tissues, provide heat, growth, and physical activity. The metabolic rate tends to vary from person to person, depending on their age, sex and lifestyle.

**MITTELSCHMERZ.** Pain associated with ovulation. It occurs usually at the time of ovulation, about halfway through the cycle. Translated, it means 'middle pain'.

**NUTRITION.** The British Society for Nutritional Medicine's definition is 'the sum of the processes involved in taking nutrients, assimilating and utilizing them'. In other words, the quality of the diet and the ability of your body to utilize the individual nutrients and so maintain health.

**OESTROGEN.** A steroid hormone which is produced in large quantities by the ovaries, and in smaller amounts by the adrenal glands. It is responsible for the development of breasts and other sexual characteristics at puberty. Oestrogen is also responsible for the production of fertile cervical mucus, the opening of the cervix, and building up of blood in the lining of the uterus, preparing for a fertilized egg.

**OVARIES.** A pair of glands situated on either side of the uterus, in which eggs and sex hormones, including oestrogen, are produced.

**OVULATION.** The release of the ripe egg (ovum) from the ovary. The two ovaries ovulate alternately every month. Occasionally, the two ovaries ovulate simultaneously, in which case the result may be twins.

**OVUM.** The egg which is released from the ovary at the time of ovulation.

**PALPITATIONS.** The heart beating too fast and sometimes irregularly.

**PITUITARY GLAND.** A small gland situated at the base of the brain, which produces many hormones, among which are those which stimulate the ovary and the thyroid.

**PRE-MENSTRUAL.** A term used to describe the time before the arrival of a period.

**PRE-MENSTRUAL SYNDROME.** This is the name given to a collection of mental and physical symptoms which manifest themselves before the onset of a period.

**PRE-MENSTRUAL TENSION.** This was the name first given to the symptoms detected before a period in 1931 by Dr Frank. Now the correct name is Pre-Menstrual Syndrome. However, many women still prefer to call the condition PMT – Pre-Menstrual Tension.

**PROGESTERONE.** A hormone secreted by the corpus luteum of the ovary during the second half of the menstrual cycle. Some studies have shown that a deficiency in progesterone may be responsible for some PMT symptoms. Progesterone is an important hormone during pregnancy.

**PROGESTOGENS.** A group of synthetic hormones, with actions similar to progesterone.

**PROLACTIN.** The hormone secreted by the pituitary gland which is involved in milk production. It is also known to affect water and mineral balance in the body, and in some women may play a part in the changes pre-menstrually.

**PROSTAGLANDINS.** Hormone-like substances found in almost every cell in the body, which are necessary for the normal function of involuntary muscles, including the heart, the uterus, blood vessels, the lungs and the intestines.

   Prostaglandins are sometimes regarded as health controllers, as they seem to play an important part in the controlling of many essential functions in the body. They do not come directly from the diet, but are made in the body itself. Because of this, the body relies on a good diet in order to produce prostaglandins. The special substances that the body needs to make these hormones are called essential fatty acids.

**SEROTONIN.** A brain chemical that influences mood.

**STEROIDS.** Substances which have a particular chemical structure in common. All the sex hormones, such as oestrogen, progesterone, etc are steroids.

**THYROID GLAND.** A gland situated in the neck, which produces the hormone thyroxine. The thyroid gland regulates metabolism.

**TRANQUILLIZERS.** A group of drugs which artificially sedate the body. They may be useful in the short term, but in the long term they can have addictive qualities.

**UTERUS (WOMB).** A sac-like organ which is located in the abdomen of a woman, and designed to hold and nourish a growing child from conception until birth.

**VAGINA.** The passage that leads from the uterus to the external genital organs.

# 2   FOOD ADDITIVES

There are many types of food additives. Most of them are denoted by a number prefixed by E. The E stands for EEC, as the European Community Regulations state that, since 1 January 1986, all foods containing additives, except for flavourings, must have an E number, or the actual name, in the list of ingredients. Some food additives are natural, vegetable-derived compounds, or even vitamins, and are perfectly harmless. However, these are not used frequently. The following additives can be associated with the exacerbation of certain medical problems:

**Azo-dyes**   E102, E104, E107, E110, E122, E123, E124, E128, E131, E132, E133, E142, E151, E154, E155, E180.
**Benzoates**   E210–E219
**Sulphur dioxide and sulphites**   E220–E227
**Nitrites and nitrates**   E249–E252
**Proprionic acid and propionates**   E280–E283
**Anti-oxidants, BHA & BHT**   E320 and E321
**Monosodium glutamate (MSG) and related compounds**   E621–E623

Many food allergy associations now give details of suppliers of foods suitable for people who suffer from allergies. Some of these are mentioned on page 227. Many supermarkets will now provide lists of their products which are free from additives, milk, wheat, eggs, etc. For those who wish to request further details, it is suggested that you contact the customer relations department of the appropriate supermarket chain.

The Ministry of Agriculture, Fisheries and Food has produced a booklet explaining what the 'E' numbers mean. There is also the excellent book 'E for Additives' by Maurice Hanssen, which is readily available. An organization called 'Foresight', The Association for the Promotion of Pre-Conceptual Care, have produced a handbag-sized booklet based on the information from the book 'E for Additives'. They have marked additive numbers with a colour code, red for danger, and they specify precisely why, orange for those additives on which conflicting reports still exist, and green for those about which there are no known side-effects. This booklet is immensely valuable as it takes the confusion out of shopping. You will find the Foresight address in Appendix 6 should you wish to obtain a copy.

# 3   ORGANIC AND SPECIALIZED FOOD SUPPLIERS

Many supermarkets are now stocking organic vegetables and grains. They are gradually expanding their ranges as and when supplies are available. The following supermarkets are included:

* Safeway's.
* Sainsbury's.
* Tesco.
* Waitrose.
* Asda.

Healthfood shops and healthfood co-ops may also stock organic produce and specialized foods.

* Cantassium Co. Ltd, 225–229 Putney Bridge Road, London SW15 2PY.
Tel: London (01) 870 0971.
Sells specialized grain products which are wheat-free etc, and supplies by mail order.

The 'Real Food Shop and Restaurant Guide', mentioned on the Reading List on page 226, has an extensive list of healthfoods and organic food suppliers.

Further information about organic foods can be obtained from The Soil Association and the Henry Doubleday Research Association. Their addresses can be found on page 229.

# 4 NUTRITIONAL SUPPLEMENT SUPPLIERS

**Retail**

| | | |
|---|---|---|
| 1. | Efamol | Boots, chemists, healthfood shops. |
| 2. | Linusit Gold | Healthfood shops. |
| 3. | Magnesium Hydroxide mixture | Boots and other chemists. |
| 4. | Optivite | Boots, chemists and healthfood shops. |
| 5. | Natural Vitamin E | Healthfood shops. |
| 6. | Vital Dophilus | Clair Laboratories Independent Distributor |

**Mail Order**

Optivite & Sugar Factor — Nature's Best Health Products, Ltd. PO Box 1, Tunbridge Wells, Kent, TN2 3EX. Tel: T.W. 0892 34143.

*Australia*

**NNFA (National Nutrition Foods Association)**
PO Box 84, Westmead, NSW 2145. Tel: 02 633 9913.
The NNFA have lists of all supplement stockists and retailers in Australia, if you have any difficulties in obtaining supplements.
Vitaglow's Premence 28 available from selected healthfood stores and pharmacists, including:
**Russells Healthfoods**, 2 Rich Street, Marrickville, NSW 2204 (tel: 569 9977). **Healthy Life** shops (head office), 100 Mount Street, North Sydney, NSW 2060 (tel: 923 4111).

*New Zealand*

**NNFA (National Nutrition Foods Association)**
c/o PO Box 820062, Auckland, New Zealand.
Again the NNFA have lists of all supplement stockists and retailers in New Zealand, if you have any difficulties in obtaining supplements.
For information on your nearest stockist of Vitaglow's Premence 28, contact: **Blackmores**, 54 Ellice Road, Glenfield, Auckland (tel: 444 3915).
* For information on where to find your local **Blackmores** and **Russells Healthfood Stores** and the products they sell, contact Angus & Robertson.

# 5 RECOMMENDED READING LIST

**NOTE**
UK, USA and A denotes the following books are available in Great Britain, United States and Australia.

### GENERAL HEALTH

1. *Diet 2000* by Dr Alan Maryon-Davis with Jane Thomas, price £1.75 (published by Pan Books). UK USA A
2. *The Food Scandal* by Caroline Walker and Geoffrey Cannon, price £3.95 (published by Century Publishing Co.) UK A
3. *Pure, White and Deadly* by Professor John Yudkin (a book about sugar), price £9.95 (published by Viking). UK A
4. *Coming off Tranquillizers* by Dr Susan Trickett, price £1.99 (published by Thorsons). UK USA A (Lothian Publishing Co.)
5. *The Better Pregnancy Diet* by Liz and Patrick Holford, price £3.95 (published by Ebury Press). UK
6. *The Migraine Revolution – The New Drug-free Solution* by Dr John Mansfield, price £3.99 (published by Thorsons). UK USA A (Lothian Publishing Co.)
7. *Conquering Cystitis* by Dr Patrick Kingsley, price £3.95 (published by Ebury Press). UK
8. *The Book of Massage*, price £6.95 (published by Ebury Press). UK
9. *Do-it-yourself Shiatsu* by W. Ohashi, price £5.50 (published by Unwin). UK
10. *Candida Albicans: Could Yeast be Your Problem?* by Leon Chaitow, price £1.95 (published by Thorsons). UK USA A (Lothian Publishing Co.)
11. *Shopping for Health* by Janette Marshall, price £3.95 (published by Penguin). UK
12. *Nutritional Medicine* by Dr Stephen Davies and Dr Alan Stewart, price £3.95 (published by Pan Books). UK A
13. *Fit for Life* by Harvey and Marilyn Diamond, price $17.50 (published by Warner Books). USA
14. *The Nutrition Detective* by Nan Kathryn Fuchs, price $16.95 (published by Jeremy P Tarcher, Inc). USA

### DIET

1. *The Allergy Diet* by Elizabeth Workman SRD, Dr John Hunter and Dr Virginia Alun Jones, price £3.95 (published by Martin Dunitz). UK USA
2. *The Candida Albicans Yeast Free Cook Book* by Pat Connolly and Associates of the Price Pottenger Nutrition Foundation, price £6.95 (published by Keats Publishing Inc). UK USA
3. *The Cranks Recipe Book* by David Canter, Hay Canter, and Daphne Swann, price £1.85 (published by Granada). UK
4. *Food Combining for Health* by Doris Grant and Jean Joice, price £5.95 (published by Thorsons). UK USA A (Lothian Publishing Co.)
5. *Food Combining Cook Book* by Edwina Lidolt, price £2.99 (published by Thorsons). UK USA A (Lothian Publishing Co.)
6. *The Food Intolerance Diet* by Elizabeth Workman SRD, Dr Virginia Alun Jones and Dr John Hunter, price £3.95 (published by Martin Dunitz). UK USA
7. *Raw Energy* by Leslie and Susannah Kenton, price £2.25 (published by Century Publishing Co.). UK A (Doubleday Publishing Co)
8. *Foresight Index Number Decoder* (Pocket Food Additive Dictionary), price £1.20, available from Foresight (address on Useful Address List page 228). UK
9. *Raw Energy Recipes* by Leslie and Susannah Kenton, price £3.95 (published by Century Publishing Co.) UK A (Doubleday Publishing Co.)

226

10. *The Real Food Shop and Restaurant Guide* by Clive Johnstone, price £3.95 (published by Ebury Press). **UK**

11. *The Sainsbury Book of Salads* by Carole Handslip, price £0.99 available from branches of Sainsbury's – excellent value. **UK**

12. *The Sainsbury Book of Wholefood Cooking* by Carole Handslip, price £0.99 available from branches of Sainsbury's – excellent value. **UK**

13. *The Reluctant Vegetarian* by Simon Hope, price £8.95 (published by William Heinemann). **UK**

14. *The Salt Free Diet Book* by Dr Graham MacGregor, price £3.95 (published by Martin Dunitz). **UK USA**

15. *Gourmet Vegetarian Cooking* by Rose Elliot, price £2.95 (published by Fontana). **UK A**

16. *Why You Don't Need Meat* by Peter Cox, price £2.50 (published by Thorsons). **UK A**

17. *Quantum Carrot, A New Concept in Small Space Organic Gardening* by Branton Kenton, price £5.95 (published by Ebury Press). **UK A**

18. *Healthy Cooking*, price £0.99 from Tesco Stores.

### STRESS

1. *Self Help for Your Nerves* by Dr Clair Weekes, price £5.95 (published by Angus & Robertson). **UK USA** (Hawthorn Publishing Co.) **A**

2. *Mind Power* by Dr Vernon Coleman, price £8.95 (published by Century Publishing Co.) **UK A**

# 6 USEFUL ADDRESSES

## GREAT BRITAIN

**British Acupuncture Register and Directory**
34 Alderney Street, London SW1V 4UE. Tel: London (071) 834 1012.

**The Council for Acupuncture**
Suite 1, 19a Cavendish Square, London W1M 9AD. Tel: London (071) 409 1440.

**Alcoholics Anonymous (AA)**
General Services Office, PO Box 1, Stonebow House, Stonebow, York YO1 2NJ. Tel: York (0904) 644026.

**Action Against Allergy**
23–24 George Street, Richmond, Surrey TW9 1JY.

**National Society for Research into Allergy**
PO Box 45, Hinkley, Leicestershire LE10 1JY.

**Anorexia and Bulimia Nervosa Association**
Tottenham Woman's and Health Centre, Annexe C, Tottenham Town Hall,
Town Hall Approach, London N15 4RX. Tel: London (081) 885 3936 (Wednesdays 6–9 pm only)

**International Federation of Aromatherapists**
4 Eastmearn Road, West Dulwich, London SE21 8HA.
Letters only enclosing an sae.

**British Pregnancy Advisory Service**
Austy Manor, Wootton Wawen, Solihull, West Midlands B95 6BX. Tel: Henley-in-Arden (05642) 3225.
*and*
7 Belgrave Road, London SW1V 1QB. Tel: London (071) 222 0985.

**Brook Advisory Centre**
Head Office, 153a East Street, Walworth, London SE17 2SD. Tel: London (081) 708 1234.

**CLEAR (Campaign for Lead Free Air)**
3 Endsleigh Street, London WC1H 0DD.    Tel: London (071) 278 9686.

**Hyperactive Children Support Group**
59 Meadowside, Angmering, Littlehampton, West Sussex BN16 4BW.
(Postal enquiries only.)

**Julia Swift Exercise Studies**
Old Slipper Baths, North Road, Brighton, Sussex.    Tel: Brighton (0273) 690016.

**ASSET**
The National Association for Health and Exercise Teachers
202 The Avenue, Kennington, Oxford OX1 5RN.    Tel: Oxford (0865) 736066.

**The Sports Council**
16 Upper Woburn Place, London WC1H 0QP.    Tel: London (071) 388 1277.

**Medau Society**
8b Robson House, East Street, Epsom, Surrey KT17 1HH.    Tel: Epsom (03727) 29056.

**Endometriosis Society**
65 Holmdene Avenue, London SE24 9LD.    Tel: London (071) 737 4764 (eve).

**Food Watch International**
Butts Pond Industrial Estate, Sturminster Newton, Dorset DT10 1AZ.   Tel: Sturminster Newton (0258) 73356.

**Foresight**
Association for the Promotion of Pre-Conceptual Care
The Old Vicarage, Church Lane, Whitney, Godalming, Surrey GU8 5PN.    Tel: Wormley (042879) 4500.

**Friends of the Earth Ltd**
26–28 Underwood Street, London N1 7JQ.    Tel: London (071) 490 1555.

**College Of Health**
14 Buckingham Street, London WC2N 6DS.    Tel: London (071) 839 2413.

**Migraine Trust**
45 Great Ormond Street, London WC1 3HD.    Tel: London (071) 278 2676.

**National Childbirth Trust**
Alexander House, Oldham, London W3 6NH.    Tel: London (081) 992 8637.

**The European School of Osteopathy**
104 Tonbridge Road, Maidstone, Kent ME16 8SL.    Tel: Maidstone (0622) 671558.

**The British School of Osteopathy**
Little John House, 1–4 Suffolk Street, London SW1 4HG.    Tel: London (071) 930 9254/8.

**Patients Association**
18 Victoria Park Square, Bethnal Green, London E2 9PF.    Tel: London (071) 981 5676.

**Action on Phobias**
c/o Shandy Mathias, 8–9 The Avenue, Eastbourne, Sussex, BN21 2YA.
Letters only enclosing an sae.

**The Women's Nutritional Advisory Service**
PO Box 268, Hove, East Sussex, BN3 1RW.    Tel: Hove (0273) 771366.

**Association for Post-Natal Illness**
7 Gowan Avenue, London SW6 6RH.    Tel: London (071) 731 4867.

**Release**
169 Commercial Street, London E16 BW.    Tel: London (071) 377 5905 and (071) 603 8654 (24-hour service).

**Samaritans**
17 Uxbridge Road, Slough SL1 1SN.    Tel: Slough (0753) 327133.

**The Shiatsu Society**
Elaine Liechti, 19 Langside Park, Kilbarchan, Renfrewshire PA10 2EP.     Tel: Kilbarchan (050 57) 4657.

**The Henry Doubleday Research Association**
Ryton Gardens, National Centre for organic gardening, Ryton on Dunsmore,
Coventry CV8 3LG.     Tel: Coventry (0203) 303517.

**The Soil Association**
86–88 Colston Street, Bristol BS1 5BB.     Tel: Bristol (0272) 290661.

Both these organizations advise on all aspects of non-chemical agriculture, give advice to amateur and professional organic growers, and have a constantly updated list of sources of organic produce.

**Ash (Action on Smoking and Health)**
5–11 Mortimer Street, London W1N 7RH.     Tel: London (071) 637 9843.

**Tranx (UK) Ltd**
National Tranquilliser Advice Centre, Registered Office, 25a Masons Avenue, Wealdstone, Harrow, Middx. HA3 5AH.     Tel: (client line) (081) 427 2065 (24-hr answering service) (081) 427 2827.

**Tranx Release, (Northampton)**
Anita Gordon, 24 Hazelwood Road, Northampton NN1 1LN.     Tel: (0604) 250976.


## AUSTRALIA

**Blackmores Limited**
23 Roseberry Street, Balgowlah, NSW 2093.     Tel: (02) 949 3177.

**Royal Society for the Welfare of Mothers and Babies**
2 Shaw Street, Petersham, NSW 2049.     Tel: (02) 568 3633.

**Childbirth Education Association of Victoria**
21 Greensborough Centre, 25 Main Street, Greensborough, Victoria 3088.

**Women's Health Advisory Service**
187 Glenmore Road, Paddington NSW 2021.     Tel: (02) 331 5014.

**Liverpool Women's Health Centre**
273 George Street, Liverpool NSW 2170.     Tel: (02) 601 3555.

**Adelaide Women's Community Health**
64 Pennington Terrace, Nth Adelaide SA 5006.     Tel: (08) 267 5366.

**PMT Relief Clinic**
Suite 6, 32 Kensington Road, Rose Park, South Australia 5067.     Tel: (08) 364 2760.


## NEW ZEALAND

**Papakura Women's Centre**
PO Box 909, Papakura, Auckland.     Tel: 299 9466.

**Whakatane Women's Collective**
PO Box 3049, Ohope.     Tel: (Whakatane) 2475.

**Health Alternative for Women**
Room 101, Cranmer Centre, PO Box 884, Christchurch.     Tel: 796 970.

**Women's Health Centre**
63 Ponsonby Road, Ponsonby, Auckland.     Tel: 764 506.

**West Auckland Women's Centre**
111 McLeod Road, Te Atatu, Auckland.     Tel: 8366 381.

**Tauranga Women's Centre**
PO Box 368, Tauranga.　　Tel: 783 530.

**The Alice Bush Family Planning Clinic**
214 Karangahape Road, Auckland.　　Tel: 775 049.

**Family Planning Clinic**
Arts Centre, 301 Montreal Street, Christchurch.　　Tel: 790 514.


### USA AND CANADA

**National Institute of Nutrition**
1565 Carling Avenue, #400, Ottawa, Ontario K12 8RI.

**The American Academy of Environmental Medicine**
PO Box 16106, Denver, Colorado, 80216.

**Optimox Inc**
PO Box 3378, Torrance, California 90510–3378.　　Tel: (800) 223 1601.


# 7　SUBSTITUTES FOR EXCLUDED FOODS

**Wheat, oats, barley, rye**　Potato flour, rice flour, soya flour, cornflour, buckwheat flour and millet flour. Usually lesser quantities of these are required. Gluten-free produce may be suitable.

**Bran (wheat)**　Soya bran and rice bran.

**Cows' milk, etc.**　Use goats' milk or ewes' milk, soya milk or non-dairy powdered milk substitute.

**Butter**　Polyunsaturate-based margarine.

**Cows' milk cheese**　Goats' or ewes' milk cheese.

**Eggs**　Duck eggs and other types of eggs can be tried.

**Yeast**　Baking powder for baking, e.g. to make soda bread.

**Sugar**　Concentrated apple juice, rice extract, artificial sweeteners, not honey.

**Corn**　Other flours, e.g. wheat, oats, soya, rice.

**Corn oil**　Sunflower seed oil, safflower seed oil, linseed oil.

**Chocolate**　Carob.

**Tea, coffee**　Herb tea, chicory and dandelion coffee.

**Vinegar**　Lemon juice.

**Potato**　Sweet potato (yams).

# 8  CHARTS AND DIARIES

SYMPTOMS

| SYMPTOMS | WEEK AFTER PERIOD (Fill in 3 days after period) | | | | WEEK BEFORE PERIOD (Fill in 2-3 days before period) | | | |
|---|---|---|---|---|---|---|---|---|
| | None | Mild | Moderate | Severe | None | Mild | Moderate | Severe |
| **PMT - A** | | | | | | | | |
| Nervous Tension | ✓ | | | | | ✓ | | |
| Mood Swings | ✓ | | | | ✓ | | | |
| Irritability | | ✓ | | | ✓ | | | |
| Anxiety | ✓ | | | | ✓ | | | |
| **PMT - H** | | | | | | | | |
| • Weight gain | | ✓ | | | | ✓ | | |
| Swelling of Extremities | | | | | | | | |
| Breast Tenderness | ✓ | | | | | | | |
| Abdominal Bloating | | | | | | | | |
| **PMT - C** | | | | | | | | |
| Headache | | ✓ | | | | ✓ | | |
| Craving for Sweets | ✓ | | | | ✓ | | | |
| Increased Appetite | ✓ | | | | | | | |
| Heart Pounding | | ✓ | | | ✓ | ✓ | | |
| Fatigue | ✓ | | | | ✓ | | | |
| Dizziness or Fainting | | ✓ | | | ✓ | | | |
| **PMT - D** | | | | | | | | |
| Depression | ✓ | | | | ✓ | | | |
| Forgetfulness | ✓ | | | | ✓ | | | |
| Crying | ✓ | | | | ✓ | | | |
| Confusion | ✓ | | | | ✓ | | | |
| Insomnia | | ✓ | | | ✓ | | | |
| **OTHER SYMPTOMS** | | | | | | | | |
| Loss of Sexual Interest | ✓ | | | | ✓ | | | |
| Disorientation | ✓ | | | | ✓ | | | |
| Clumsiness | ✓ | | | | ✓ | | | |
| Tremors/Shakes | | | | | | | | |
| Thoughts of Suicide | ✓ | | | | ✓ | | | |
| Agoraphobia | ✓ | | | | | | | |
| Increased Physical Activity | ✓ | | | | | | | |
| Heavy/Aching Legs | | ✓ | | | | ✓ | | |
| Generalized Aches | ✓ | | | | | ✓ | | |
| Bad Breath | ✓ | | | | ✓ | | | |
| Sensitivity to Music/Light | | ✓ | | | ✓ | | | |
| Excessive Thirst | ✓ | | | | | ✓ | | |

Do you have any other PRE-MENSTRUAL SYMPTOMS not listed above?

1. _____

2. _____

3. _____

4. _____

•5.   How much weight do you gain before your period? _____

# MENSTRUAL SYMPTOMATOLOGY DIARY

Month: April

### GRADING OF MENSES

| | |
|---|---|
| 0-none | 3-heavy |
| 1-slight | 4-heavy and clots |
| 2-moderate | |

### GRADING OF SYMPTOMS (COMPLAINTS)

0-none
1-mild-present but does not interfere with activities
2-moderate-present and interferes with activities but not disabling
3-severe-disabling. Unable to function.

| Day of cycle | 1 | 2 | 3 | 4 | 5 | 6 | 7 | 8 | 9 | 10 | 11 | 12 | 13 | 14 | 15 | 16 | 17 | 18 | 19 | 20 | 21 | 22 | 23 | 24 | 25 | 26 | 27 | 28 |
|---|---|---|---|---|---|---|---|---|---|---|---|---|---|---|---|---|---|---|---|---|---|---|---|---|---|---|---|---|
| Date | 23 | 24 | 25 | 26 | 27 | 28 | 29 | 30 | 1 | 2 | 3 | 4 | 5 | 6 | 7 | 8 | 9 | 10 | 11 | 12 | 13 | 14 | 15 | 16 | 17 | 18 | 19 | 20 |
| Period | 1 | 4 | 3 | 2 | 1 | 0 | 0 | 0 | 0 | 0 | 0 | 0 | 0 | 0 | 0 | 0 | 0 | 0 | 0 | 0 | 0 | 0 | 0 | 0 | 0 | 0 | 0 | 0 |

### PMT-A

| | | | | | | | | | | | | | | | | | | | | | | | | | | | | |
|---|---|---|---|---|---|---|---|---|---|---|---|---|---|---|---|---|---|---|---|---|---|---|---|---|---|---|---|---|
| Nervous tension | 1 | 0 | 0 | 0 | 0 | 0 | 0 | 0 | 0 | 0 | 0 | 0 | 0 | 0 | 0 | 0 | 0 | 0 | 0 | 0 | 0 | 0 | 0 | 0 | 1 | 1 | 0 | 1 |
| Mood swings | 0 | 0 | 0 | 0 | 0 | 0 | 0 | 0 | 0 | 0 | 0 | 0 | 0 | 0 | 0 | 0 | 0 | 0 | 0 | 0 | 0 | 0 | 0 | 0 | 0 | 0 | 0 | 1 |
| Irritability | 0 | 0 | 0 | 0 | 0 | 0 | 0 | 0 | 0 | 0 | 0 | 1 | 0 | 0 | 0 | 0 | 0 | 0 | 1 | 0 | 1 | 0 | 1 | 0 | 0 | 0 | 1 | 1 |
| Anxiety | 1 | 0 | 0 | 0 | 0 | 0 | 0 | 0 | 0 | 0 | 0 | 0 | 0 | 0 | 0 | 0 | 0 | 0 | 0 | 0 | 0 | 0 | 0 | 0 | 0 | 0 | 0 | 0 |

### PMT-H

| | | | | | | | | | | | | | | | | | | | | | | | | | | | | |
|---|---|---|---|---|---|---|---|---|---|---|---|---|---|---|---|---|---|---|---|---|---|---|---|---|---|---|---|---|
| Weight gain | 0 | 0 | 0 | 1 | 0 | 1 | 1 | 0 | 0 | 0 | 0 | 0 | 0 | 1 | 1 | 0 | 0 | 0 | 0 | 0 | 1 | 0 | 1 | 0 | 1 | 1 | 0 | 0 |
| Swelling of extremities | 1 | 1 | 1 | 1 | 1 | 1 | 1 | 1 | 1 | 0 | 0 | 1 | 1 | 1 | 1 | 1 | 0 | 0 | 1 | 1 | 1 | 2 | 1 | 1 | 1 | 1 | | |
| Breast tenderness | 1 | 1 | 1 | 0 | 1 | 1 | 0 | 0 | 0 | 0 | 0 | 0 | 1 | 0 | 0 | 0 | 0 | 1 | 1 | 1 | 1 | 1 | 1 | | | | | |
| Abdominal bloating | 1 | 1 | 1 | 1 | 1 | 1 | 1 | 1 | 0 | 0 | 1 | 1 | 1 | 1 | 0 | 1 | 1 | 1 | 1 | 1 | 1 | 1 | 0 | 0 | | | | |

### PMT-C

| | | | | | | | | | | | | | | | | | | | | | | | | | | | | |
|---|---|---|---|---|---|---|---|---|---|---|---|---|---|---|---|---|---|---|---|---|---|---|---|---|---|---|---|---|
| Headache | 1 | 1 | 2 | 1 | 1 | 1 | 0 | 0 | 0 | 1 | 0 | 1 | 0 | 0 | 0 | 0 | 1 | 0 | 0 | 0 | 0 | 0 | 0 | 0 | 1 | | | |
| Craving for sweets | 0 | 0 | 0 | 0 | 0 | 0 | 0 | 0 | 0 | 0 | 0 | 0 | 0 | 0 | 0 | 0 | 0 | 0 | 0 | 0 | 1 | 0 | 1 | 0 | 0 | 0 | | |
| Increased appetite | 0 | 0 | 0 | 0 | 0 | 0 | 0 | 0 | 0 | 0 | 0 | 0 | 0 | 0 | 0 | 0 | 0 | 0 | 0 | 1 | 0 | 0 | 0 | 0 | | | | |
| Heart pounding | 0 | 1 | 1 | 1 | 0 | 0 | 0 | 0 | 0 | 0 | 0 | 0 | 0 | 0 | 0 | 0 | 0 | 0 | 0 | 0 | 0 | 1 | 0 | 0 | | | | |
| Fatigue | 1 | 1 | 1 | 0 | 0 | 0 | 0 | 0 | 0 | 0 | 0 | 0 | 0 | 0 | 1 | 0 | 1 | 1 | 0 | 0 | 0 | 0 | 0 | 1 | | | | |
| Dizziness or faintness | 0 | 2 | 1 | 1 | 1 | 0 | 0 | 0 | 1 | 1 | 1 | 0 | 0 | 0 | 0 | 0 | 1 | 0 | 0 | 1 | 0 | 0 | 0 | 0 | | | | |

### PMT-D

| | | | | | | | | | | | | | | | | | | | | | | | | | | | | |
|---|---|---|---|---|---|---|---|---|---|---|---|---|---|---|---|---|---|---|---|---|---|---|---|---|---|---|---|---|
| Depression | 0 | 0 | 0 | 0 | 0 | 0 | 0 | 0 | 0 | 0 | 0 | 0 | 0 | 1 | 0 | 0 | 0 | 0 | 0 | 0 | 0 | 0 | 0 | 0 | 0 | 1 | | |
| Forgetfulness | 0 | 0 | 0 | 0 | 0 | 0 | 0 | 0 | 0 | 0 | 0 | 1 | 0 | 0 | 0 | 0 | 0 | 0 | 0 | 0 | 0 | 0 | 0 | 0 | | | | |
| Crying | 0 | 0 | 0 | 0 | 0 | 0 | 0 | 0 | 0 | 0 | 0 | 1 | 0 | 0 | 0 | 0 | 0 | 0 | 0 | 0 | 0 | 0 | 0 | 0 | | | | |
| Confusion | 0 | 0 | 0 | 0 | 0 | 0 | 0 | 0 | 0 | 0 | 0 | 0 | 0 | 0 | 0 | 0 | 0 | 0 | 0 | 0 | 0 | 0 | 0 | 0 | | | | |
| Insomnia | 0 | 0 | 0 | 1 | 0 | 0 | 0 | 0 | 0 | 0 | 0 | 0 | 0 | 0 | 0 | 0 | 0 | 0 | 0 | 0 | 0 | 0 | 0 | 0 | | | | |

### PAIN

| | | | | | | | | | | | | | | | | | | | | | | | | | | | | |
|---|---|---|---|---|---|---|---|---|---|---|---|---|---|---|---|---|---|---|---|---|---|---|---|---|---|---|---|---|
| Cramps (low abdominal) | 1 | 1 | 1 | 0 | 0 | 1 | 1 | 0 | 0 | 0 | 0 | 0 | 0 | 1 | 1 | 0 | 0 | 0 | 0 | 1 | 0 | 1 | 0 | 0 | 0 | | | |
| Backache | 1 | 0 | 1 | 0 | 1 | 1 | 1 | 1 | 1 | 0 | 0 | 0 | 0 | 1 | 0 | 0 | 0 | 0 | 1 | 0 | 0 | 1 | 0 | | | | | |
| General aches/pains | 0 | 0 | 0 | 1 | 1 | 0 | 0 | 1 | 1 | 0 | 1 | 1 | 0 | 1 | 0 | 0 | 1 | 1 | 1 | 0 | 1 | | | | | | | |

NOTES:

# MENSTRUAL SYMPTOMATOLOGY DIARY

Month: May

### GRADING OF MENSES

| | |
|---|---|
| 0-none | 3-heavy |
| 1-slight | 4-heavy and clots |
| 2-moderate | |

### GRADING OF SYMPTOMS (COMPLAINTS)

0-none
1-mild-present but does not interfere with activities
2-moderate-present and interferes with activities but not disabling
3-severe-disabling. Unable to function.

| Day of cycle | 1 | 2 | 3 | 4 | 5 | 6 | | | | | | | | | | | | | | | | | | | | | | | |
|---|---|---|---|---|---|---|---|---|---|---|---|---|---|---|---|---|---|---|---|---|---|---|---|---|---|---|---|---|---|
| Date | 21 | 22 | 23 | 24 | 25 | 26 | | | | | | | | | | | | | | | | | | | | | | | |
| Period | 2 | 4 | 2 | 1 | 1 | 0 | | | | | | | | | | | | | | | | | | | | | | | |

**PMT-A**

| Nervous tension | 0 | 1 | 1 | 1 | 0 | 0 | | | | | | | | | | | | | | | | | | | | | | | |
|---|---|---|---|---|---|---|---|---|---|---|---|---|---|---|---|---|---|---|---|---|---|---|---|---|---|---|---|---|---|
| Mood swings | 2 | 1 | 0 | 0 | 0 | 0 | | | | | | | | | | | | | | | | | | | | | | | |
| Irritability | 2 | 2 | 0 | 0 | 0 | 0 | | | | | | | | | | | | | | | | | | | | | | | |
| Anxiety | 0 | 1 | 1 | 1 | 0 | 0 | | | | | | | | | | | | | | | | | | | | | | | |

**PMT-H**

| Weight gain | 1 | 0 | 1 | 0 | 0 | 0 | | | | | | | | | | | | | | | | | | | | | | | |
|---|---|---|---|---|---|---|---|---|---|---|---|---|---|---|---|---|---|---|---|---|---|---|---|---|---|---|---|---|---|
| Swelling of extremities | 2 | 1 | 2 | 0 | 1 | 1 | | | | | | | | | | | | | | | | | | | | | | | |
| Breast tenderness | 1 | 1 | 1 | 1 | 0 | 1 | | | | | | | | | | | | | | | | | | | | | | | |
| Abdominal bloating | 0 | 0 | 1 | 0 | 0 | 0 | | | | | | | | | | | | | | | | | | | | | | | |

**PMT-C**

| Headache | 0 | 2 | 1 | 0 | 0 | 1 | | | | | | | | | | | | | | | | | | | | | | | |
|---|---|---|---|---|---|---|---|---|---|---|---|---|---|---|---|---|---|---|---|---|---|---|---|---|---|---|---|---|---|
| Craving for sweets | 0 | 0 | 0 | 1 | 0 | 1 | | | | | | | | | | | | | | | | | | | | | | | |
| Increased appetite | 0 | 0 | 0 | 0 | 1 | 1 | | | | | | | | | | | | | | | | | | | | | | | |
| Heart pounding | 0 | 0 | 1 | 1 | 1 | 1 | | | | | | | | | | | | | | | | | | | | | | | |
| Fatigue | 0 | 1 | 0 | 0 | 0 | 0 | | | | | | | | | | | | | | | | | | | | | | | |
| Dizziness or faintness | 0 | 0 | 0 | 0 | 0 | 0 | | | | | | | | | | | | | | | | | | | | | | | |

**PMT-D**

| Depression | 0 | 0 | 0 | 0 | 0 | 0 | | | | | | | | | | | | | | | | | | | | | | | |
|---|---|---|---|---|---|---|---|---|---|---|---|---|---|---|---|---|---|---|---|---|---|---|---|---|---|---|---|---|---|
| Forgetfulness | 0 | 0 | 0 | 0 | 0 | 0 | | | | | | | | | | | | | | | | | | | | | | | |
| Crying | 0 | 0 | 0 | 0 | 0 | 0 | | | | | | | | | | | | | | | | | | | | | | | |
| Confusion | 0 | 0 | 0 | 0 | 0 | 0 | | | | | | | | | | | | | | | | | | | | | | | |
| Insomnia | 0 | 0 | 0 | 0 | 0 | 0 | | | | | | | | | | | | | | | | | | | | | | | |

**PAIN**

| Cramps (low abdominal) | 1 | 0 | 1 | 0 | 0 | 0 | | | | | | | | | | | | | | | | | | | | | | | |
|---|---|---|---|---|---|---|---|---|---|---|---|---|---|---|---|---|---|---|---|---|---|---|---|---|---|---|---|---|---|
| Backache | 1 | 0 | 0 | 0 | 1 | 0 | | | | | | | | | | | | | | | | | | | | | | | |
| General aches/pains | 1 | 0 | 0 | 0 | 0 | 1 | | | | | | | | | | | | | | | | | | | | | | | |

NOTES:

233

# 9 REFERENCES

### Chapter 1

1. Green R., Dalton K. The Pre-Menstrual Syndrome. British Medical Journal. May 9, 1953. P1007–1014.
2. Abraham G.E. Nutrition and the Pre-Menstrual Tension Syndromes. Journal of Applied Nutrition. 36:103–124. 1984.
3. Morton J. H., Additon H., Addison R.G., Hunt L., Sullivan J.J. A clinical study of Pre-Menstrual Tension. A.M.J.Obstet.Gynecol. 55:1182–1191. 1953.

### Chapter 2

1. Abraham G.E. Management of the Pre-Menstrual Tension Syndromes: Rationale for a Nutritional Approach. In: A Year in Nutritional Medicine, Second Edition 1986. Ed. by Bland J. Keats Publishing, Inc. New Canaan, Conrecticut: 125–166. 1986.
2. Munday M.R., Brush M.G., Taylor R.W. Correlation between Progesterone, Oestradiol and Aldosterone Levels in the Pre-Menstrual Syndrome. Clinical Endocrinology. 14:1–9. 1981.
3. Watts J.F.F., Butt W.P., Logan Edwards R., Holder G. Hormonal Studies in Women with Pre-Menstrual Tension. British Journal of Obstetrics and Gynaecology. 92:247–255. 1985.
4. Dalton M.E. Sex Hormone-Binding Globulin Concentrations in Women with Severe Pre-Menstrual Syndrome. Post-Graduate Medical Journal. 57:560–561. 1981.

### Chapter 3

1. Moos R.H. Typology of Menstrual Cycle Symptoms. American Journal of Obstet.Gynec. 103:390–402. 1969.

### Chapter 4

1. Dalton K. Pre-Menstrual Syndrome and Progesterone Therapy. Second Edition. William Heinemann Medical Books Limited London. 1984.
2. Hargrove J.T., Abraham G.E. The Incidence of Pre-Menstrual Tension in a Gynaecologic Clinic. The Journal of Reproductive Medicine. 27:721–724. 1982.
3. Hargrove J.T., Abraham G.E. The Ubiquitousness of Pre-Menstrual Tension in a Gynaecologic Practice. The Journal of Reproductive Medicine. 28:435–437. 1983.

### Chapter 5

1. Yudkin J. Pure White and Deadly. Viking Press. London. 1986.
2. Royal College of General Practitioners. Alcohol – A Balanced View. Report from General Practice 24. RCGP London. 1986.
3. Drug Abuse Briefing. Institute for the Study of Drug Dependents. London. 1986.
4. Abraham G.E. Nutrition and the Pre-Menstrual Tension Syndromes. Journal of Applied Nutrition. 36:103–124. 1984.
5. Ashton C.H. Caffeine and Health. The British Medical Journal. 295:1293–4. 1987.

### Chapter 6

1. Boyle C.A. et al. Caffeine Consumption and Fibrocystic Breast Disease: A Case-Control Epidemiologic Study. JNCI. 72:1015–1019. 1984.
2. O'Brien P.M.S, Selby C., Symonds E.N. Progesterone, Fluid and Electrolytes in Pre-Menstrual Syndrome. The British Medical Journal. 10 May 1980: 1161–1163.
3. MacGregor G.A. et al. Is 'Idiopathic' Oedema Idiopathic. The Lancet 1:397–400. 1979.
4. O'Brien P.M.S., Selby C., Symonds E.M. Progesterone, Fluid and Electrolytes in Pre-menstrual Syndrome. The British Medical Journal. 280:1161–3. 1980.

### Chapter 7

1. Yudin J. Pure White and Deadly. Viking Press. London. 1986.
2. Morton J.H., Additon H., Addison R.G., Hunt L., Sullivan J.J. A clinical study of Pre-Menstrual Tension. A.M.J.Obstet.Gynecol. 55:1182–1191. 1953.

**Chapter 8**
1.  Abraham G.E. Nutrition and the Pre-Menstrual Tension Syndromes. Journal of Applied Nutrition. 36:103–124. 1984.
2.  Dalton K. Pre-Menstrual Syndrome and Progesterone Therapy. Second Edition. William Heinemann Medical Books Limited London. 1984.


**Chapter 9**
1.  Dalton K. Pre-Menstrual Syndrome and Progesterone Therapy. Second Edition. William Heinemann Medical Books Limited London. 1984.


**Chapter 10**
1.  Pre-Menstrual Syndrome – Proceedings for Workshop held at the Royal College of Obstetricians and Gynaecologists. London, 2nd December 1982. Ed. Taylor. R.W. Medical News – Tribune Limited. London. 1983.
2.  Sampson J.A. Pre-Menstrual Syndrome: A Double-Blind Control Trial of Progesterone and Placebo. British Journal of Psychiatry. 135:209–215. 1979.
3.  Dennerstein L., et al. Progesterone and the Pre-Menstrual Syndrome: A Double-Blind Cross Over Trial. British Medical Journal. 290:1617–1621. 1985.
4.  Magos A., Studd J. Progesterone and the Pre-Menstrual Syndrome: A Double-Blind Cross Over Trial. British Medical Journal. 291:213–214. 1985.
5.  O'Brien P.M.S. The Pre-Menstrual Syndrome: A Review of the Present Status of Therapy. Drugs 24:140–151. 1982.


**Chapter 11**
1.  Modern Nutrition in Health and Disease. Ed: Goodhart R.S., Shils M.E. Sixth edition Lea and Febiter, Philadelphia. 1980.
2.  Nutritional Medicine. Davies S., Stewart A. Pan Books London. 1987.
3.  Lewis J., Buss D.H. Trace Nutrients 5. Minerals and Vitamins in the British Household Food Supply. British Journal of Nutrition. 60:413–424. 1988.
4.  Spring J.A., Robertson J., Buss D.H. British Journal of Nutrition. 41:487–493. 1979.


**Chapter 12**
1.  Piesse. J.W. Nutrition Factors in the Pre-Menstrual Syndrome. International Clinical Nutrition Review. 4:54–81. 1984.
2.  Hargrove J.T., Abraham G.E. Effect of Vitamin B6 on Infertility in Women with Pre-Menstrual Syndrome. Infertility 2:315–322. 1979.
3.  Abraham G.E., Hargrove J.T. The Effect of Vitamin B6 on Pre-Menstrual Symptomatology in Women with Pre-Menstrual Syndrome: A Double-Blind Cross Over Study. Infertility. 3:155–165. 1980.
4.  Gunn A.D.G. Vitamin B6 and the Pre-Menstrual Syndrome. In Vitamins-Nutrients as Therapeutic Agents. Ed: Hanck A., Hornig D. Hans Huber Publishers. Bern. 1985. P213–224.
5.  Stokes J., Mendels J. Pyridoxine and Pre-Menstrual Tension. The Lancet 1:1177–1178. 1972.
6.  Abraham G.E. Magnesium Deficiency in Pre-Menstrual Tension. Magnesium Bulletin 1:68–73. 1982.
7.  Abraham G.E., Lubran M.M. Serum and Red Cell Magnesium levels in patients with Pre-Menstrual Tension. The American Journal of Clinical Nutrition. 34:2364–2366. 1981.
8.  Sherwood R.A., Rocks B.F., Stewart A., Saxton R.S. Magnesium in the Pre-Menstrual Syndrome. Ann. Clin. Biochem. 23:667–670. 1986.
9.  Pre-Menstrual Tension: An Invitation a Symposium. Ed. Abraham G.E. Journal of Reproductive Medicine. 28:7 & 8:433–538. 1983.
10. Fushs N., Hakim M., Abraham G.E. The Effect of a Nutritional Supplement, Optivite, for Women with Pre-Menstrual Tension Syndromes. 1. Effect of Blood Chemistry and Serum Steroid levels during the mid-luteal phase. The Journal of Applied Nutrition. 37:1–11. 1986.
11. Chakmakjian Z.H., Higgins C.E., Abraham G.E. The Effect of a Nutritional Supplement, Optivite, for Women, on Pre-Menstrual Tension Syndromes: 2. The effect of Symptomatology, using a Double-Blind Cross-Over Design. The Journal of Applied Nutrition. 37:12–17. 1986.

**12.** London, R.S. et al. The Effect of Alpha-Tocopherol on Pre-Menstrual Symptomatology: A Double-Blind Study. Journal of the American College of Nutrition. 2:115–122. 1983.

**13.** London, R.S. et al. The Effect of Alpha-Tocopherol on Pre-Menstrual Symptomatology: A Double-Blind Study 2. Endocrine correlates. Journal of the American College of Nutrition. 3:351–356. 1984.

**14.** O'Brien P.M.S. Pre-Menstrual Syndrome. Blackwell Scientific Publications, Oxford, 1987.

**15.** Stewart A.A. Rational Approach to Treating Pre-Menstrual Syndrome. WNAS publication, 1989.

**16.** Stewart A. Clinical and Biochemical Effects of Nutritional Supplementation on the Pre-Menstrual Syndrome. The Journal of Reproductive Medicine. 32:435–441. 1987.

**17.** Boyd E.M.F. et al. The effect of a low fat, high complex-carbohydrate diet on symptoms of cyclical mastopathy. Lancet. 2:128–132. 1988.

### Chapter 13

**1.** Yudkin J. Pure White and Deadly. Viking Press, London. 1986.

**2.** Royal College of General Practitioners. Alcohol – A Balanced View. Report from General Practice, 24. RCGP. London 1986.

**3.** Health Education Council. Thats The Limit – Booklet. HEC, 78 New Oxford Street, London EC1A1AH.

**4.** Nutritional Medicine by Dr Stephen Davies and Dr Alan Stewart. Pan Books. 1987.

**5.** Which? Troubled Waters, Which? November 1986. P494–497.

**6.** Spring J.A., Robertson J., Buss D.H. Trace Nutrients 3. Magnesium, Copper, Zinc, Vitamin B6, Vitamin B12 and Folic Acid in the British Household Food Supply. Br.J.Nutr. 41:487–493. 1979.

**7.** Victor B.S., Greden J.F., and Lubetsky, M. Somatic Manifestations of Caffeinism. J.Clin Psychiat. 42:185–8. 1981.

**8.** Disler P.B. et al. The Effects of Tea on Iron Absorption. Gut 18:193–200. 1975.

**9.** Tonkin S.Y. Vitamins and Oral Contraceptives. In Vitamins in Human Biology in Medicine. Ed: Briggs M.H. CRC Press, Boca Raton, Florida. P29–64. 1981.

**10.** Walters A.H., Fletcher, J.R., Law S.J. Nitrate in Vegetables: Estimation by HPLC. Nutrition and Health. 4:141–149. 1986.

**11.** Mount J.L. The Food and Health of Western Man. Charles Knight & Co Ltd, London. 1975.

**12.** The Booker Health Report – A Survey of Vitamin and Mineral Intakes within Certain Population Groups. Booker Health Foods. 1986.

### Chapter 18

**1.** Chuong C.J., Coulam C.B., Kao P.C., Bergstalh J., Go V.L.W. Neuropeptide levels in Pre-menstrual Syndrome. Fertility and Sterility. 44:760–765. 1985.

# INDEX

Aches, 22, 79
Acne/skin problems, 22, 139
Acupuncture and acupressure, 209–11
Adrenal glands, 19, 20, 49, 126
Adrenaline, 28, 56
Aggression, 30, 92, 124
Agoraphobia, 22, 36, 79, 82–3, 195
Alcohol, 57, 98, 99, 102, 106, 109–10, 124, 125, 126, 131, 138, 161
Aldosterone, 49
Allergies, 96
    foods, to, 163–70, 172–3, 195, 230
Aluminium, 106, 107
Amino acids, 99–100
Anaemia, 57, 130, 139
Animal fats, 28
Ankles, swollen, 22
Antacids, 107
Anti-depressants, 13, 113
Antibiotics, 104, 116
Anxiety, 22, 26, 28–48, 101, 107, 108, 114, 124, 139
Appetite, increase of, 56, 139
Arthritis, 96
Asthma, 22, 96

Backache, 22
Bloating, 22, 26, 49–55, 115, 139, 162, 167
Blood pressure, 96
Boils, 22
Bran, 128
Breakfast recipes, 180–1
Breast size, increase in, 49
Breast tenderness, 12, 22, 24, 26, 33, 49–55, 107, 114, 115, 139, 159, 172
Breath, bad, 22, 79

Caffeine, 29, 57, 97, 102, 107–8, 159
Calcium, 106, 109, 128, 146–7, 159
Cancer, 96, 97, 98, 100
Carbohydrates, 122–3
Case histories
    Anita Walker, 61, 63, 72–8, 91–2, 94, 95, 117, 151, 169
    Geraldine Ellis, 57–62, 81–2, 92, 116, 134, 169–70
    Jane Moor, 83–8, 116, 214, 217–18
    Nadine Morris, 43–8, 218–19
    Pauline Solent, 31–7, 78, 118
    Rebecca Harley, 53–5, 135
    Ruth Sears, 37–43, 95, 117–18
    Sally Noone, 67–72, 94
    Sandra Patterson, 134–5
    Vivienne Tanner, 52–3, 115
Cervical mucus, 15, 16

Cervix, 15
Charts, 150–6, 232
Chocolate, 29, 56, 57, 159
Cholesterol levels, 104, 122
Chromium, 102, 128, 131–2, 147, 170
Clumsiness, 22, 79, 80
Coffee, 29, 57, 97, 102, 107–8, 124, 130, 131, 138, 157, 159
Cola-based drinks, 29, 57, 105, 159
Confusion, 22, 27, 139
Constipation, 22, 162, 164
Contraceptive pill, 25, 99, 117, 125, 131, 169
    PMT treated with, 99, 113, 116–17
Copper, 102, 128, 131
    as toxin, 106
Cracked mouth or lips, 167, 170, 175
Cramp, 22
Cravings, food, 12, 22, 26, 56–63, 92, 131, 139, 170
Crying, 22, 27, 64–78, 139
Cystitis, 22, 167

Dairy products, 138, 159
Depression, 22, 27, 64–78, 101, 114, 124, 139, 162, 167, 195, 199
    post-natal, 58, 213
Diabetes, 96
Diarrhoea, 22, 162, 195
Diary, keeping, 153, 155–6, 232–3
Diet, 13, 25, 27, 85, 88, 103–5, 113–15, 121–3
    agricultural chemicals, 97, 98
    allergies, 163–70, 172–3, 195
    cholesterol, 104, 122
    complex carbohydrates, 115, 122
    cooking processes, 102
    fats, 121–2
    fatty acids, 122, 171
    fibre, 28, 100, 103, 123
    food additives, 98, 107, 224
    frozen foods, 103
    nitrates, 98
    organic produce, 104, 106, 140, 224
    pesticides, 97, 98
    phosphorus, 97
    PMT A, 28–9, 36, 41, 44, 46, 139
    PMT C, 56–7, 61, 139
    PMT D, 68, 70, 72, 74, 76, 139
    PMT H, 50, 51–2, 53, 139
    polyunsaturated fats, 148
    progesterone levels, 18
    proteins, 121
    refined and processed foods, 50, 97, 99, 101, 103, 107, 129, 137–8

237

saturated fats, 97, 99, 100, 103, 104, 115
substitutes for excluded foods, 230
vegetarian and vegan, 104, 109, 126, 140, 162
*see also* Minerals; Nutrition; Vitamins
Dinner recipes, 186–92
Disorientation, 22, 79
Diuretics, 113, 115, 130, 131
Dizziness, 22, 26, 57, 139
Dopamine, 28
Driving ability, effect of PMT, 94–5
Drug treatment, 99, 113, 115–16, 178
    meat from treated animals, 104
    withdrawal from, 118–19, 178
Drugs, social stimulants, 57

Eczema, 22, 96, 122
Electroconvulsive therapy (ECT), 33
Endometrium, 15
Environmental pollution, 97, 103, 105–6
Evening primrose oil, 113, 114, 122, 134
Exercise, 138–9, 196, 198–205

Facial hair, 24
Fainting, 22, 26, 57, 139
Fallopian tubes, 15
Fatigue, 12, 22, 26, 56–63, 139, 162
Fish, 104
Fluid retention, 12, 49–50, 123, 129–30, 160
Forgetfulness, 22, 27, 139

Glucose, 122–3
Grains, allergy to, 163–7

Hayfever, 22, 96
Headaches, 22, 24, 26, 56–63, 139, 170
Heart disease, 96, 97, 100, 104, 107
Heart pounding, 22, 26, 57, 139
Hives, 22
Hormones, 19
    aldosterone, 49
beta-endorphin, 198–9
    depression affected by, 65
    hormonal treatments, 13, 33, 113, 116–18, 212
    *see also* oestrogen; progesterone
Hostility, 22
Hyperactivity, 96, 107
Hyperventilation, 29
Hypoglycaemia, 56
Hypothalmus, 19, 20

Insomnia, 22, 27, 107, 108, 139, 195
Iron, 57, 101, 108–9, 126, 128, 130, 132–3, 134, 144–5, 162, 170–1
Irritability, 22, 26, 28–48, 124, 139
Irritable bowel syndrome, 44, 48, 195

Joints, painful, 22

Lead, as toxin, 105–6, 107
Legs, aching or restless, 22, 79
Light, sensitivity to, 22, 79
Lunch recipes, 186–92

Magnesium, 28, 57, 101, 106, 109, 113, 114, 128–9, 130, 132–3, 135, 142–3, 214
Meat, 98, 103–4, 140
Mefenamic acid, 115
Memory loss, 124
Menopause, 14, 212–13
Menstrual cycle, 14–20
Mental illness, 96
Metabolism, 120–1, 122
Migraine, 22, 170, 195
Minerals, 57, 99–100, 101–2, 128–33
    alcohol consumption, 109
    blocks to absorption, 108–9
    contraceptive pill, effect of, 99
    nutritional treatment, 113–14
    physical signs of deficiency, 174, 175
    supplements, 41, 174, 176–8
    toxic, 105–6
Mood swings, 22, 26, 28, 139, 195

Nervous tension, 12, 22, 26, 28, 107, 139, 195
Nipples, discharge from, 24
Nitrates, 98, 105
Noise, sensitivity to, 22, 79
Noradrenaline, 28
Nutrition, 120–36
    absorption of nutrients blocked, 101, 105
    menstrual cycle, effect on, 18–19
    side effects of treatment by, 114
    and stress, 195
    supplements, suppliers of, 225
    treatment programmes, 113–15, 119, 137–78
    *see also* Diet

Oestrogen, 16, 29, 126
    effect on nervous system, 18–19
    high levels of, 12, 28
    implants, 113, 117
    increased sensitivity to, 28
    lead, affected by, 64
    PMT A, 28
    PMT D, 64
    PMT H, 49
Osteopathy, 208–9
Osteoporosis, 20
Ovaries, 15
Ovulation, 15–16, 21

Pain killing drugs, 113
Periods
    heavy, 12, 24, 139, 170–1, 214

irregular, 24, 214
period pains, 23, 213–14
Phosphorus, 128
Physical activity, increased, 22, 79
Pituitary gland, 16, 19, 20, 135
Potassium, 128, 129–30
Pre-Menstrual Syndrome (PMT)
  A (anxiety), 26, 28–48, 64, 139, 152–3, 159
  C (craving), 26, 39, 56–63, 139, 153
  D (depression), 27, 39, 64–78, 134, 139, 153, 159
  H (hydration), 26, 49–55, 135, 139, 153
  contributing factors, 24–7
  dietary and nutritional treatments, 114–15
  disease state leading to, 121
  drug treatments, 115–16, 118–19
  hormonal treatments, 116–18
  social implications, 91–5
  symptoms, 21, 22, 26–7
  treatments for, 112–19
  twentieth-century lifestyle, 96–7
Progesterone, 16, 18, 126
  effect on nervous system, 18–19
  low levels of, 12, 18
  PMT H, 49
  treatment with, 12, 113, 116
Pyridoxine, 109, 113–14

Recipes
  breakfast, 180–1
  lunch and dinner, 186–92
  salad and salad dressings, 183–6
  soups, 181–3
  sweets, 192–4
Relaxation, 196–7, 199, 200, 206–7
Restlessness, 22

Salad and salad dressings, 183–6
Salt, 50, 97, 129, 138, 160
Sedatives, 99, 113, 118–19
Selenium, 102, 128
Serotonin, 28, 49
Sex drive, 79, 80–2
Shiatsu, 210–11
Smoking, 57, 98, 102, 125, 126, 138, 139, 161
Social stimulants, 57
Sodium, 128, 129–30
Soup recipes, 181–3
Sterilization, 214–15
Stress, 20, 25, 27, 56, 67, 73, 97, 173–4, 195–7
Sugar, 50, 56, 57, 68, 97, 99, 100, 103, 104–5, 122, 137–8, 160–1
Suicidal feelings, 22, 64–78, 79

Sweets, recipes for, 192–4
Swollen extremities, 22, 26, 49, 50, 139

Tannin, 108
Tea, 29, 57, 97, 101, 102, 108–9, 124, 130, 131, 138, 157, 159
Thiamin, 109
Thirst, excessive, 22, 79
Thrush, 41, 74, 99, 130, 134, 167, 169–70
Thyroid, 19, 20, 57, 135
Toxins, 105–7
Tranquillizers, 13, 99, 115–16, 118–19
Tremors, 22, 79

Ulcers, mouth, 22, 162, 175
Uterus (womb), 15

Vaginal
  discharge, 24
  soreness or irritation, 24
Vegetarian diet, 104
Violent feelings, 30, 88–90, 92
Vitamins, 123–7
  A, 123, 124
  B group, 12, 20, 28, 64, 100–1, 106, 109, 113–14, 123, 124–6, 131, 132–3, 135, 142, 168, 195, 214
  C, 106, 123, 126–7, 132–3, 145–6, 214
  D, 109, 123, 127
  E, 113, 114, 123, 127, 146, 214
  K, 123
  alcohol consumption, 109
  bioflavonoids, 127, 214
  contraceptive pill, effect of, 99
  deficiencies, 99–100
  nutritional treatment, 113–14
  physical signs of deficiency, 174, 175
  supplements, 41, 174, 176–8

Water, 123
  pollutants in, 98, 105, 106
Weight, 51–2
  and depression, 64
  gain, 12, 22, 24, 26, 49–55, 73–4, 139
  heavy periods, 214
  loss, 24
Wind, 22, 162, 167
Women's Nutritional Advisory Service, 10
Work, productivity and efficiency at, 93–4

Yeast, allergy to, 67–8, 167–70

Zinc, 20, 102, 106, 108, 109, 128, 131, 132–3, 135, 143–4, 162, 171

"PMT – A Self Help Guide". A 30 minute VHS video for PMT sufferers and Health Care Professionals, covering:

- The extent of the problem
- How mood swings, irritability, depression, fatigue, bloating and other symptoms can damage relationships, family life and work
- A review of treatments available
- Why experts recommend the nutritional approach to treating PMT as the most effective first line treatment
- An outline of the nutritional recommendations for sufferers

ORDER FORM

Post coupon (and payment) to: WNAS Video Unit, PO Box 268, Hove, East Sussex BN3 1RW.

Please send me _____ copies of PMT – A Self Help Guide price £8.99 each (inc. VAT and postage & packing). I enclose a cheque/postal order for £ _____ payable to the WNAS Video Unit, or please debit my Barclaycard / Access account number

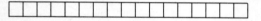

Expiry date _____ £ _____ Signature _____

Or you can phone 0273 771366 direct quoting your Barclaycard / Access account number.

Videos should arrive within 28 days of receipt of your order.

AVAILABLE FROM SEPTEMBER 1990

The Women's Nutritional Advisory Service
BEAT PMT COOKBOOK
by Maryon Stewart
with Sarah Tooley

Over 100 tempting new recipes based on the bestselling *Beat PMT Through Diet*
Paperback price £5.99

Available from your local bookshop or by mail order from Murlyn Book Services, PO Box 50, Harlow, Essex CM17 0DZ at £6.49 (£5.99 + p&p) each. Send a postal order/cheque made out to *Murlyn Book Services* or quote your Visa/Access number.

Or you can phone 0279 635377 quoting your Visa/Access number.